The Pathology and Pharmacology of Mental Illness

Mark Wilbourn

Sylvia Prosser

First published in 2003 by:
Nelson Thornes Ltd
Delta Place
27 Bath Road
CHELTENHAM
GL53 7TH
United Kingdom

03 04 05 06 07 / 10 9 8 7 6 5 4 3 2 1

A catalogue record for this book is available from the British Library

ISBN 0-7487-5321-4

Page Make-up by Acorn Bookwork

Printed and bound in Croatia by Zrinski

The   ogy

Contents

Preface

This book has been written particularly for mental health workers of all disciplines who need to understand the physical causes of problems commonly encountered by their clients and the principles of action of the major groups of drugs used to treat some of their problems. The authors make no claim to be pharmacologists. They have worked from the perspective of being college lecturers and health professionals, who know from experience some of the areas of difficulty for health students trying to apply knowledge, derived from biomedical science, to their practice with clients. Readers who may not possess a sophisticated background in biochemistry and neuroscience may encounter difficulty in understanding some facets of the basis of mental illness and how drugs work. The authors hope that this book will help readers to obtain and apply knowledge to their practice in a useful way. For this reason, the format of the book includes clinical examples, key points and self-test material, also references to some of the current literature and electronic sources. The growing concern with herbal and alternative treatments has led to the inclusion where possible of information concerning these forms of treatment. We hope that readers find it helpful.

Mark Wilbourn MSc; BSc (Hons); CertEd; RMN
Senior Lecturer, Professional Lead for Mental Health, Faculty of Health, Canterbury Christ Church University College, UK

Sylvia Prosser PhD; MSc; BEd (Hons) RGN
Principal Lecturer, Biomedical Sciences, Faculty of Health, Canterbury Christ Church University College, UK

INTRODUCTION

1

This book has been written for health professionals who work with clients with mental health problems. Such professionals may represent a range of disciplines, such as nurses, occupational therapists, social workers, probation officers or officers working in custodial institutions. In this book, the term 'mental health professional' is used to encompass all of these occupational groups. In some contexts, such as the sections in this chapter related to administration of medication, a role is taken by a specific health professional, who is usually a nurse. In such sections, the relevant health professional will be named specifically.

MEDICATION AND THE PATIENT WITH MENTAL HEALTH PROBLEMS

Communication within and between cells

The complex functions of the nervous system are possible because some cells have developed and specialised in their ability to communicate. All cells have systems by which they are able to make contact locally and with distant tissues (Figure 1.1). It is important to understand normal physiology in order to appreciate altered physiology and the action of medication.

Inter- and intracellular communication

Cellular communication occurs between the cell and the extracellular fluid by means of the structure of the cell membrane. Substances capable of combining with the phospholipid cell membrane may diffuse inside and alter the chemical balance and activity within the cell. Other substances may be actively transported into the cell via active transport mechanisms. Small channels between cells enable messenger chemicals to pass from one cell to another within a tissue and thus enable one cell to influence the functioning of another. Hormones may bind to receptor molecules on the cell's surface and alter the level of the cell's functioning (Table 1.1). As a molecule binds with a cell surface receptor, a change in an internal substance called a G-protein stimulates an alteration in the internal chemical structure and the creation of

Autocrine communication	Chemicals secreted within the cell by that cell alter or modify cellular functioning
Paracrine communication	Chemicals secreted within one cell enter a neighbouring cell and modify its function
Endocrine communication	Hormones from distant cells bind with target cell receptors and influence functioning

Table 1.1

Summary of cellular communication systems.

Chemical communication systems enable communication to take place within and between cells

Figure 1.1

Structure of a cell

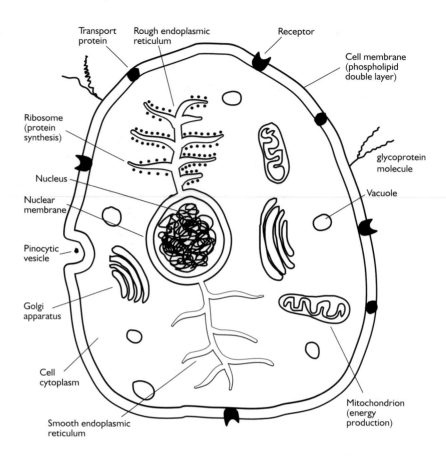

substances called second messengers that influence the way in which the cell functions.

Control systems: the neuroendocrine systems

Within the body, two major communication systems exist. One system involves nerve transmission, the other the production of hormones.

Nerve transmission: the rapid-response system

Within the nervous system, communication is effected via neurones, which are specialised communication cells. As has been discussed above, cell membranes are capable of interaction with their external environment. Neurones are cells that have become supersensitive to stimulus (or in other words, are irritable) and have adapted their cell membranes so that when a stimulus such as an alteration in the chemical constituents of the extracellular fluid occurs, minute channels in the cell membrane actively transport positively charged ions into that cell, as is shown in Figure 1.2.

Cells are organised into blocks of tissue that have assumed a particular function. To illustrate this, it is useful to consider our development from an immobile single-celled organism into a complex

(i) A neurone is a cell specifically developed for communication
     It has the characteristic of IRRITABILITY

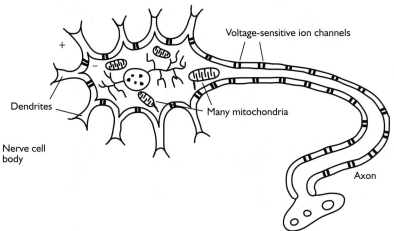

(ii) At rest, there are more positively charged ions outside the nerve cell.
      The neurone cytoplasm is relatively negatively charged.

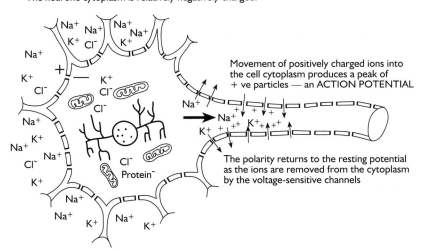

Figure 1.2

Generation of an action potential
(a) 'Resting' nerve cell. There are more positively charged ions outside the cell than inside. The resting potential of the cell interior can therefore be considered as negative and is measured as a negative value of millivolts.
(b) A stimulus produces a change in the cell's action potential. Local voltage-sensitive channels allow positively charged ions such as sodium (Na^+), potassium (K^+) and calcium (Ca^{++}) to enter the cell. The electrical potential within the cell begins to rise from the negative resting values, and changes from a negative to a positive state. Once more, this potential for activity can be measured in millivolts. At this point, the cell membrane is said to be polarised.
(c) The voltage-sensitive channels pump the positively charged ions from the nerve cell cytoplasm and return them to the extracellular fluid. The negative resting potential is restored and the cell is said to be depolarised.
(d) This process is repeated by each voltage-sensitive channel along the length of the axon of the neurone. The effect is that of a wave of positively charged particles travelling along the neurone.
(e) The action potential reaches the terminal part of the neurone. A neurotransmitter substance is released from store and diffuses into the extracellular fluid of the synapse. As it combines with the cell membrane of the neighbouring dendrite, the process of generating an action potential in the next neurone is begun.

creature able to move purposefully, coordinate activity, experience emotion, react and reason (Figure 1.3).

The nervous system has finally become so complex and important that there is an array of subsystems that contribute to normal neural functioning. In overview, there are three subsystems, the central nervous system (CNS), comprising the brain and spinal cord; the peripheral nervous system, which comprises the nerves which ramify through the tissues (such as muscles, motor nerves, joint and tendon receptors) to bring movement under control of the brain, and the autonomic nervous system which is responsible for all of the maintenance of functioning of the vital systems, for example breathing, control of heart rate, maintenance of blood pressure. When mental health problems arise, imbal-

Figure 1.3

Development of areas of functioning within the nervous system (a) A simple organism consisting of a number of cells acquires the ability to move. Irritability enables the organism to twitch out of the way of danger.

(b) The organism evolves into a more complex creature. Nerves and muscle groups have developed, which need some basic form of control. An example is a centipede, which needs to be able to co-ordinate its many legs so that they work in a synchronised manner. Such coordination is undertaken by the spinal cord, in just the same way that a newborn baby's 'stepping' reflex is the result of spinal cord activity.

(c) The organism needs to be able to get out of trouble, and also to compete for food or a mate. An area of nervous tissue able to respond to challenge or danger is needed. The limbic system develops at the head of the spinal cord and the amygdala and hippocampus modulate primitive drives and emotions such as fear, aggression and long-term memory.

(d) The organism grows yet more complex and needs to be able to balance and to synchronise the activity of a range of muscle groups so as to move in a synchronised, smooth way. The cerebellum evolves. Special senses such as sight and hearing develop to enable maximum interpretation of the environment.

(e) Life has now become so complicated that the creature needs to be able to think, weigh up options and predict results. The cerebral cortex evolves and is localised into specific areas of function.

(a)

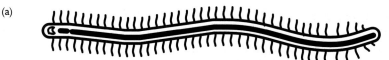

As multicelled organisms evolved, there was a need to undertake and coordinate complex movement

The precursor of a spinal cord, and then a cerebellum developed. Newborn babies make stepping movements when held via a **spinal reflex**.

(b)

Once coordinated movement was possible, the animal developed centres for behaviour and emotions (e.g. fear, aggression, mating). The increasingly complex organism also needed physiological control mechanisms

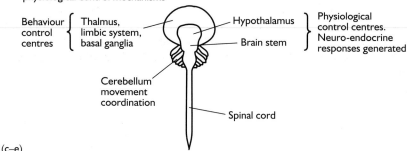

(c–e)

Increasingly sophisticated functions (e.g. speech, hearing, integration of inputs and outputs, cognitive activity) create the need for large areas of brain tissue. The cerebral cortex develops.

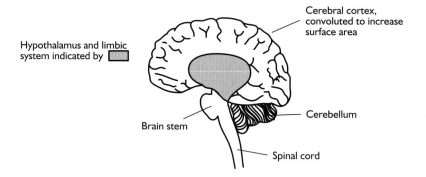

ances of these systems may result. For example, panic attacks are commonly associated with rapid pulse rate or hyperventilation – inappropriately rapid rates of breathing. Clients taking neuroleptic drugs to control cognitive disorders such as schizophrenia may suffer problems with control and regulation of movement and be seen to have tremor (shaking of the limbs) or ataxia (staggering gait). When functioning normally, the neural responses enable the body to react according to need within fractions of a second.

Nerves are cells that have specialised in rapid communication. They can be found throughout the body.

Endocrine responses

The other mechanism is the endocrine system, which enables tissues to communicate with distant structures via the production of hormones. The blocks of tissue that produce hormones are called endocrine glands

– these have a good vasculature and secrete their products directly into the bloodstream. Hormone systems tend to work more slowly than the nervous mechanisms and operate by means of feedback mechanisms, so a reduction in circulating hormone levels is detected by receptors and the endocrine gland is stimulated to secrete more of its product into the plasma. If the hormone levels in the blood become elevated, this is detected and the endocrine gland activity is suppressed until the plasma concentration returns to the required level. A reduction below normal of the hormone level causes stimulation of the gland to increase output. Cells controlled by a given hormone have specific receptors. In addition to the flexibility of the endocrine to alter the output of hormone according to demand, cells are able to down- or upregulate the number of the hormone receptors according to the levels of circulating hormone (Figure 1.4)

(a)

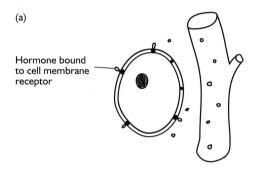

Hormone bound to cell membrane receptor

Normal levels of hormone in plasma: hormones diffuse to extracellular fluid and bind to receptors on cell membrane, causing changes to occur within the cell

Figure 1.4

Cellular regulation of hormone receptors in response to plasma levels

(b)

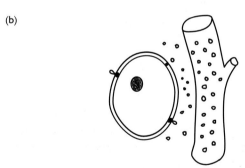

Too much hormone in plasma: cell membrane receptors shut down, providing fewer receptor sites for hormone binding

(c)

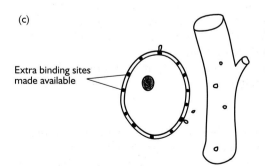

Extra binding sites made available

Low levels of hormone in plasma: cell membrane receptors open up, providing maximum levels of binding sites for available hormone molecules

In contrast to the virtually instantaneous response time of the nervous system, endocrine responses occur within hours, days or a period of weeks. The endocrine system organises tissue reactions to support the changes made by the nervous system. Stress is a good example of combined response between the nervous and endocrine system. For a further explanation of the stress response, see Chapter 2.

Key point ▶

> The endocrine system provides a slower communication system that acts in conjunction with the nervous system.

Figure 1.5

Example of a negative feedback mechanism

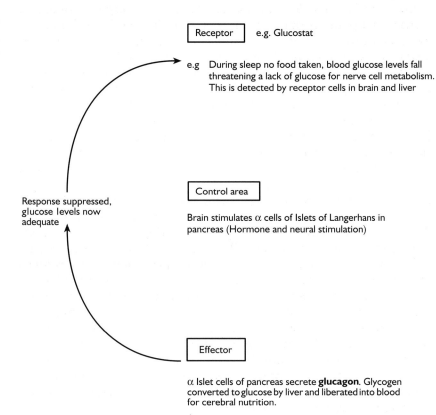

Receptor   e.g. Glucostat

e.g During sleep no food taken, blood glucose levels fall threatening a lack of glucose for nerve cell metabolism. This is detected by receptor cells in brain and liver

Response suppressed, glucose levels now adequate

Control area

Brain stimulates α cells of Islets of Langerhans in pancreas (Hormone and neural stimulation)

Effector

α Islet cells of pancreas secrete **glucagon**. Glycogen converted to glucose by liver and liberated into blood for cerebral nutrition.

Key point ▶

> The close link between mind and body means that mental ill-health commonly produces associated physical symptoms

Biology of emotions

The understanding of the physical basis of behaviour and emotions was initially obtained by observing people with known brain injuries who eventually died, following which their brain could be examined in detail. Many illuminating histories exist, some of which are discussed by Sacks (1995), who describes the classical example of Phileas Gage, a 19th century railway worker who sustained a brain injury to his temporal lobe following an accident with a rod that penetrated his brain from below his cheek when an explosive he was positioning detonated prematurely. Although he was lucky to survive, the result was disastrous for Gage, who changed from being an industrious, responsible person to become unemployable because of a personality change that produced childish, irresponsible behaviour and an inability to put plans into logical operation – a distinct disadvantage in a worker who needed to use explosives!

Over the last few decades, the development of magnetic resonance imaging and positron emission tomography techniques have allowed the living brain to be studied in a non-invasive manner so as to examine anatomical structures, biochemical composition, blood flow and oxygen uptake. It has thus been possible to learn that behaviour and emotions are governed by specific areas of the brain. The orbitofrontal cortex (the area in the base of the brain just above the eyes) seems to play a parti-cular role in the assessment of the personal consequences of action. This is the area of the cerebral cortex that was damaged in Phileas Gage's case, which explains his subsequent lack of success as a railway explo-sives worker. This area of the cerebral cortex seems to be associated with self-protecting inhibitions and emotional responses to pain. Following damage, the individual can consider theoretical problems but cannot plan in order to translate an idea into action. People with damage to these areas of the brain have reduced inhibitions and inability to protect themselves from harm. The prefrontal lobes of the brain seem to have a role in dealing with both anxiety and frustration. It was found that, if the nerve fibres to these areas of the brain were divided surgi-cally in a prefrontal lobotomy, antisocial behaviour or disabling anxiety could be controlled. Unfortunately, the after-effects of this procedure were that the patient suffered personality changes of irresponsibility, childishness, difficulty in transforming ideas into action and loss of normal emotional responses, and the procedure became discredited. Normally, emotional responses have a role in decision-making and experiential learning, and these had been lost as a result of surgical interference with the prefrontal lobes.

The amygdala has been observed to become more active when the subject is experiencing anxiety. Within the amygdala there are neurones with receptors that readily combine with molecules of benzodiazepine tranquilliser (see Chapter 2). It is therefore likely that there are natural 'tranquillity molecules', which work at these sites and limit arousal. Neurones within the amygdala also combine readily with cholecysto-kinin, another transmitter substance. Cholecystokinin, when used experimentally, produces sensations of fear and anxiety, and events generating sensations of fear are known to produce increased levels of cholecystokinin in the amygdala (Carlson, 2001). When experimental volunteers are faced with a difficult task or lists of threatening words, scanning studies have shown that blood flow increases through the bilateral structures of the amygdala. Patients with damage to the amygdala have a decreased experience of fear and their emotions do not have the usual effect upon memory formation.

The cingulate gyrus appears to function as an interface between decision-making structures within the frontal cortex and brain mechanisms controlling movement. This part of the brain communicates with other parts of the limbic system and areas within the frontal cortex, thus acting rather as an emotional 'junction box'. Electrical stimulation here influences the emotions and damage to this structure causes the individual to become silent and immobile. Interestingly, it has been suggested that extroverts have greater levels of activity of their cingulate gyri. Introverts have increased activation of the prefrontal cortex, which would produce behavioural inhibition (Johnson *et al.*, 1999).

Specific hormones and neurones have also been found to govern behaviour; for example, aggressive behaviour is suppressed by serotonergic neurones (Carlson, 2001). Alcohol interacts with serotonin, which helps to explain why alcohol ingestion is often a contributory factor when fights take place. Androgens also tend to produce aggressive behaviour.

Key point ▶

> Behaviour is governed by specific areas of the brain and the presence of particular synaptic neurotransmitters. Modern techniques for investigating the living brain have made a significant contribution to the biology of emotions.

PRINCIPLES OF PHARMACOLOGY: DRUGS AND THE BODY

When a client needs pharmacological treatment for a particular mental health problem, the medication given often works by influencing the cellular mechanisms explained above. In this section, general factors relating to drugs and their interaction with the body are considered.

It must be remembered that drugs are treated by the body as if they are unwanted substances – in other words, as if they were poisons. So, although drugs are prescribed to have a specific effect upon the body (the effect of drugs upon physiological functioning is termed **pharmacodynamics**), from the moment of entry of drugs into the body, the body will have an effect upon the medication. This handling of drugs by the body is called **pharmacokinetics**. Relevant principles of pharmacodynamics are considered in the chapters discussing specific mental health disorders and treatment, and relate to the selection of the correct drug for the client. Some key ideas that it is important to understand in relation to pharmacokinetics will now be reviewed.

When a client is given medication, it is important that s/he receives enough of the drug to achieve a predictable treatment for the problem while avoiding too great a concentration, which would result in a toxic effect. When giving medication to clients, nurses must ensure that the client receives the correct drug in the correct amount by the correct route at the correct time. The aim is to achieve an adequate concentration of the drug in the tissues to be treated so as to achieve a therapeutic effect.

◀ **Key point**

> The body handles drugs as if they were poisons to be excreted. This must be taken into account when medication is prescribed.

The 'correct route': routes of administration

As already explained, in order to have an effect, drugs need to enter the tissues to be treated, and they usually arrive there via the bloodstream. The most familiar route by which drugs enter the body is via the mouth and the alimentary tract – the **enteral** route. Some substances are given by rectal suppositories, in which case the active ingredient is presented within a vehicle, such as glycerine, that melts within the warmth of the body, releasing the active agent, which then diffuses into the bloodstream via the walls of the blood vessels lining the rectum. Drugs may also be administered **parenterally**, for example by being injected subcutaneously or intramuscularly. Muscle is well supplied with blood vessels so when a client receives an intramuscular injection the medication diffuses from the muscle vasculature into the bloodstream. Medication can also be administered intravenously or it can be delivered into the bloodstream via the nasal or respiratory mucosa in the form of a nasal spray or respiratory inhaler. As a rule, when drugs are directly introduced into the circulation, the therapeutic effect is obtained more rapidly, as the mechanisms by which digestion and absorption occur are bypassed.

◀ **Key point**

> In order to exert a therapeutic effect, drugs must be delivered to the target tissue. The circulation is an important transport mechanism for medication.

For most people, the most acceptable way of taking medication is via tablets or capsules taken by mouth. Uncoated tablets begin to be broken down in the mouth and stomach. Some substances may be inactivated by gastric juices or may damage the gastric mucosa, so are produced in an **enteric-coated** format. In this case, the coating remains intact in the stomach but is broken down in the duodenum, thus releasing the product into the small intestine. A more long-lasting effect may be obtained by the use of **sustained-release** oral preparations in which the drug is presented in a format of mini capsules within a gelatine outer capsule. This format provides a supply of the product in small quantities over a longer period of time as the units are gradually broken down over a lengthened time span.

Some clients may find it difficult to remember to take oral medication or may for some reason find it unacceptable to take tablets. In cases where severe mental illness uncontrolled by medication is likely to result in psychosis, a better therapeutic effect from medication may be obtained by injection. To avoid the discomfort of frequent injections, the product may be given as a **depot injection**. In this case the drug is presented in the form of microcrystals or suspended in some other medium such as oil, wax or a synthetic substance, which results in a slow liberation of the active drug into the subcutaneous or intramuscular vasculature.

Apart from the acceptability or otherwise to the client, use of the correct route is important in ensuring that the dose prescribed is what the patient actually receives. The prescriber must be able to predict that a given amount of a preparation will result in a specific concentration of the drug in the client's CNS or other body tissue. The use of a different route or preparation format will alter the concentration of the preparation from that which the prescriber originally predicted, so the result to the client could be either an inadequate dose to obtain a therapeutic effect, or toxicity. It is important to remember this when clients have difficulty in taking medication: opening capsules or crushing up coated tablets is likely to alter the **bioavailability**, so the amount of the drug available to treat the disorder becomes altered and the therapeutic concentration may be lost: in this situation, the nurse has administered the medication but, in so doing, has ceased to participate in the effective treatment of the client, because the client has not received the drug in a valid format.

Key point ▶

> Differing routes of administration influence the bioavailability of drugs.

When a client is being treated for a mental health problem, the medication used will usually need to be transported to the CNS via the circulatory system. The cardiovascular system is a major transport medium, and most drugs are carried either attached to plasma proteins or dissolved in the plasma. In order to enter the target organ where treatment is needed, plasma-bound drugs must detach from the protein molecule and then diffuse from the plasma into the extracellular fluid and from there into the cells to be treated. Some drug interactions occur because of competition for space on carrier proteins. For instance, a client may be receiving treatment with a particular drug that is being carried on a particular part of a plasma protein molecule. If that client is then prescribed another agent that is also carried in the same way, the second drug may displace the first and alter the bioavailability, thus producing an increased, or possibly toxic, effect. Therefore, when multiple prescription is needed, it is important that the prescriber checks for potential drug interactions.

◀ **Key point**

> Because of the way molecules of drugs are carried within the circulation, addition of further types of medication may alter bioavailability.

The 'blood–brain barrier'

There is a particular challenge related to the use of drugs to treat disorders of the brain, because the CNS is protected by the blood–brain barrier. In order for chemicals to affect the brain, they need to get into brain cells or into the extracellular fluid surrounding them. It has been seen that neurones are irritable, that is, they respond by producing action potentials when chemical changes occur within the extracellular compartment. It would be undesirable for action potentials to be generated whenever a chemical change took place somewhere within the bloodstream, so the CNS is protected by a barrier that serves to isolate the brain and spinal cord from such potential disruption. The cells of the walls of the blood vessels within the brain are more tightly joined together than in the other blood vessels of the body. This results in the vessels being much less permeable; therefore it is far more difficult for substances to leave the bloodstream and enter the brain. A limited number of substances are able to pass freely from the bloodstream into the tissues of the brain. Some substances, such as glucose, which the

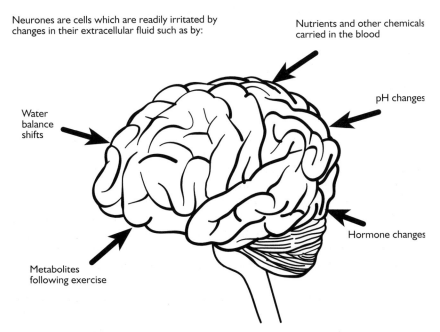

Neurones are cells which are readily irritated by changes in their extracellular fluid such as by:

Nutrients and other chemicals carried in the blood

pH changes

Water balance shifts

Hormone changes

Metabolites following exercise

Protection of the brain achieved by:
Relatively impermeable walls of cerebral blood vessels.
Cellular pumps to control access of molecules from/to brain.
Lipid layer surrounding neurones

Figure 1.6

The blood–brain barrier

brain requires for energy, are actively transported across the capillary walls; cerebral metabolites are transported in the opposite direction from the brain to the bloodstream, and are removed from the CNS accordingly.

In order to be able to enter the brain or to influence the workings of neurones, drugs need to be able to pass through the blood–brain barrier. For this to be possible, they must have a particular chemical formulation.

Key point ▶

> Drugs used to treat mental health problems must be able to cross the blood–brain barrier so as to enter the CNS.

HOW THE BODY DEALS WITH DRUGS

First pass metabolism

Just as food must undergo digestion and absorption before it can travel in the blood, so medication taken by mouth is changed chemically during its passage through the alimentary system. A certain amount of the drug is usually inactivated as a result of passage through the stomach and intestines, which is termed first pass metabolism. First pass metabolism means that some of the prescribed dose will never exert a therapeutic effect on the tissues because it has been broken down prematurely. Drug regimes must take into account this 'wastage' to ensure that the plasma and target tissue concentration is in fact sufficient to provide effective treatment. This is the reason why the dose of a drug taken by mouth is usually greater than when the same substance is administered via another route.

Drug excretion

In order for the chemistry of the body to be kept within normal limits, the excretory mechanisms must constantly remove potentially dangerous toxins and metabolites. Two major systems are responsible for this excretion: the liver and the kidneys.

Hepatic excretion

The liver is the major organ which breaks down toxins and prepares them for excretion. Alteration of drugs by the liver takes place in two stages. In **stage 1 metabolism**, the molecules of the drug are rearranged by the liver and intermediate metabolites are created. These generally still have some pharmacological effect, although they may differ in character from the original preparation. When a new drug is developed, the effect and duration of the metabolites has to be taken into account by the pharmaceutical company to ensure that the correct therapeutic concentration is achieved.

In **stage 2 metabolism**, the liver completes the breakdown of the metabolites into a form that can be excreted. The drug has now completely lost its pharmaceutical effect and has been converted into a water-soluble form that can be removed from the body either via the kidneys in the urine or, as in the case of some anaesthetic gases, in the expired air or, in other cases, in the faeces via the biliary system and the gastrointestinal tract. If a client has impaired liver or kidney function, the ability to remove drugs from the body is reduced and toxicity may result from dosages that would be normal for other people. In older people, liver or kidney function may be less effective, so these clients may be prescribed smaller doses or require frequent checks of drug plasma levels to ensure that the concentration remains at therapeutic levels. (See the section below discussing therapeutic levels.)

An important example of the effect of a drug metabolite may be seen in paracetamol overdosage. In therapeutic doses, when the drug is taken according to the manufacturer's recommendations to obtain analgesia, paracetamol is gradually converted into a metabolite that, although potentially harmful, is made safe by being combined by the liver with glutamate, an enzyme. The liver has only limited stores of glutamate, so, when a significant overdose is taken that produces plasma levels of around 1.32 mmol/l, large amounts of a toxic metabolite are produced. In this circumstance, the stores of protective glutamate are used up and the liver cells are damaged irretrievably.

Therapeutic levels

The constant action of the liver and kidneys in treating medication as a poison to be removed from the body means that achieving the correct concentration of a drug being given to a client can be likened to trying to fill a bath with the taps running and the plug out. When a client is first started on a medication, no treatment will occur until the plasma levels reach a sufficient concentration to enable the drug to diffuse into the tissues to be treated and to achieve a sufficient concentration in the tissues to treat the pathophysiology causing the problem. In order to build up to a therapeutic level, the rate of entry of the drug into the body must exceed the speed at which the excretory mechanisms dismantle and remove the chemical. So, when commencing a prescription, the dose must be of sufficient size and frequency to build up to and then maintain the correct concentration in the plasma and the tissues. Some drugs, notably those acting on the CNS, take additional time to reach their target organ and so take even longer to begin to exert a therapeutic effect. At this stage, it is understandable that the client may lose faith in the treatment, consider that it is not working and discontinue the medication before it has even begun to work. If this mechanism is understood by those caring for the patient, a suitable explanation of why it takes time for the medication to work may help to encourage the client to persist with medication and receive effective treatment. Figure 1.6 shows how therapeutic levels build up, and then 'wash out' when treatment is discontinued. It is important to realise that the doses of some drugs, such as lithium (see Chapter 3) need to be

Figure 1.7

The development of therapeutic levels in the plasma.

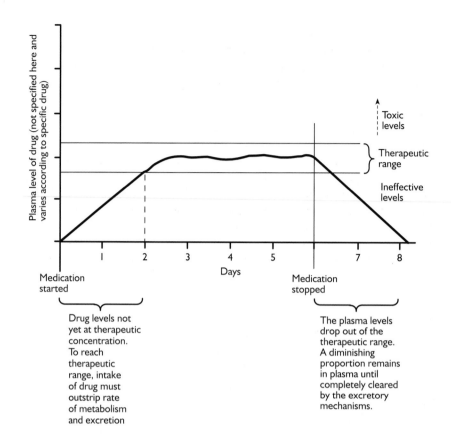

Plasma level of drug (not specified here and varies according to specific drug)

Toxic levels

Therapeutic range

Ineffective levels

Days

Medication started

Medication stopped

Drug levels not yet at therapeutic concentration. To reach therapeutic range, intake of drug must outstrip rate of metabolism and excretion

The plasma levels drop out of the therapeutic range. A diminishing proportion remains in plasma until completely cleared by the excretory mechanisms.

finely controlled as the **therapeutic margin** is very narrow: a dose suffi-cient to treat the client's symptoms is very close to that which produces toxic effects. In such cases, the client needs regular monitoring of the plasma levels to ensure that the dose remains effective but not toxic.

Key point ▶

> Time is needed for a therapeutic drug dosage to build up. This is because of the effect of the excretory mechanisms upon the plasma levels.

At the end of treatment, when the prescription is discontinued, it may be important to remember that, even though the client has stopped taking the medication, the drug concentration will drop gradually as the process of breakdown and elimination continues.

Changing medication

As can be seen in Figure 1.7, once the client stops taking the prescription, there is a gradual reduction in the plasma levels as the excretory mechanisms gradually reduce the plasma concentration. It is important to remember that, should a client require a change in medication, if the new agent is incompatible with the original preparation, it may be necessary for a time lapse to occur between successive prescriptions. This is particularly the case when antidepressant treatment is changed (see Chapter 3), as the different groups of antidepressants tend to interact adversely together.

Dosage

In order to obtain sufficient concentration of the drug within the bloodstream and therefore to the CNS, the client must receive the **correct dose** of medication. As has been explained above, a whole range of factors influence the maintenance of the therapeutic levels. Thus, the route of administration, the format of the preparation and the frequency of administration all influence the therapeutic levels. Some drugs induce tolerance, which means that, if usage is prolonged, an increased dose is needed to achieve the same pharmacological effect. This occurs notably when opioid analgesia is prescribed. The development of tolerance is a different mechanism from drug dependency (see Chapter 7).

Specificity

One more concept that needs to be explored when considering the principles of pharmacology is that of **specificity**. When a chemical enters the body and is transported in the circulation, it may come in contact with many different organs and tissues. In order to achieve the desired treatment, the drug must enter the correct target tissue and must combine with receptors or the cell membrane or cross the cell wall in some other way. If medication is being prescribed for one problem, the client requires that problem, and that problem only, to be remedied. A client being treated for schizophrenia may receive treatment that affects the parts of the brain which govern mood and behaviour (see Chapter 5). Unfortunately, the hypothalamus is a near neighbour of these structures and can be affected by some neuroleptic medication. This can cause changes to the endocrine system, which is controlled by hypothalamic releasing factors. The ideal is for a drug to combine specifically with the tissues to be treated and no other, but this is not always easily achieved.

> Ideally, a drug has a specific action upon the target tissues. This depends upon the molecular compatibility between the drug and the receptors on the target tissue cells.

◄ *Key point*

Alternative remedies

Many people choose to take alternative remedies. Some herbal and nutritional substances are pharmacologically active and clients find them helpful. It is important for mental health professionals to remember that the use of such remedies may interact with prescribed medication. Questions such as 'Are you taking any medicines from your doctor?'

may not elicit the information that the person is using an alternative remedy, which may be important to acknowledge within an overall treatment plan. In some cases, the client may need to choose between the prescribed medication and the alternative remedy because a combination of the two substances will produce an adverse reaction. Apart from the fact that the client may have derived benefit from use of the alternative substance, there are issues about being 'in control' and being able to obtain alternative substances without an appointment with a medical practitioner that make their use attractive to some people.

The extent to which compounds that enhance mood – such as strong coffee, tea, chocolate, cola drinks, alcohol in all its forms and tobacco – should be viewed as 'medication' is debatable; this would complicate the client's personal life as well as their mental health care considerably. For example, nicotine induces certain enzymes and so may cause subtle changes in the effect of medication. Some clients think that herbal remedies are inherently safer than pharmacological substances but they need to realise that compounds such as opium, heroin and cocaine are derived from herbal sources and that these are not necessarily harmless in their actions. It is important therefore that clients feel that they can trust mental health professionals sufficiently to discuss the relative safety and effectiveness of alternative substances and to engage in shared control in relation to the choice and use of medication. An interesting series of vignettes illustrating the use of alternative substances by mentally ill clients is presented in Yager *et al.*, 1999.

Box 1.1

The placebo effect

The human brain is extremely sensitive to stimuli and suggestion. Most of us have experienced a headache that we think we have treated with minor analgesics such as aspirin or paracetamol. The headache resolves, but then we find that the painkillers are still on the table – we may have experienced a 'placebo effect'! Some clients, such as those with minor anxiety, may be more susceptible to the placebo effect than others whose belief systems have been altered by mental illness.

Overdosage

The main specific features of overdosage of a given drug are indicated in the appropriate section. To avoid duplication, the major principles are indicated below.

It is important to consider the possibility of drug overdosage when working with clients with mental health problems. The overdose may be accidental or deliberate and aspects of the treatment plan will need to be reviewed accordingly. General principles of physical care for a patient who has overdosed start with ascertaining the time at which the overdose was taken. If this was recent, then the drug may still be in the stomach. It is important to know what has been taken, so any containers and substances should be kept to help identify the nature of the overdose. If the client vomits, it is useful to keep a specimen as it may be used for chemical analysis to identify the substances taken, also to record that the client has vomited. It is useful to refer to a pharmaceutical formulary such as the British National Formulary (BNF) for specific detail related to the drug taken in overdose so as to know what to look for when assessing the client. Help lines such as the Guy's Poisons Centre offer 24-hour expert advice to assist in the management of poisoning.

In some cases, when the overdose has been taken within the last few hours, it is necessary to remove the drug that has not been absorbed from the stomach. This is usually done by inducing emesis (vomiting) or performing a gastric lavage (stomach washout) in a hospital with acute medical back-up facilities. Use of stomach washout as a deterrent against future overdosage has little validity, so the procedure should only be performed under appropriate medical direction when indicated by the client's physical condition.

General principles of caring for a client include assessing consciousness levels; checking airway, respiratory rate and skin colour; checking blood pressure and pulse. The specific effects of a given drug taken in overdose can be seen in a current formulary, but the effects can often be grouped as shown in Table 1.2.

Table 1.2

Common features of poisoning and principles of treatment

Consciousness	May be depressed – in this case check and maintain the airway to ensure the client is able to breathe. Convulsive seizures may be a feature Some drugs cause hyperactivity; this does not necessarily mean that the overdose is trivial
Breathing	Some drugs cause respiratory depression in overdose. Is the client breathing normally? Is airway support needed?
Cardiovascular system	Some drugs cause cardiac arrhythmias. Is the pulse regular? Some overdoses cause hyper- or hypotension: what is the blood pressure?
Gastrointestinal system	Some drugs in overdose cause diarrhoea and/or vomiting sufficient to produce hypovolaemic shock. Check upper airway for obstruction by vomit, check blood pressure for shock
The main immediate killers are cardiovascular and respiratory dysfunction and cerebral seizures. Check for these first!	**Antidotes are relatively few and medication is usually aimed at reducing absorption or increasing elimination from the gastrointestinal tract**

It is important to remember that an overdose may involve a range of substances and that this will complicate the client's condition. The effects of the individual substances ingested may be altered by interactions between the various substances. Alcohol may have been taken and this will complicate the picture further.

DRUGS, THE LAW AND MENTAL HEALTH CARE

In this part of the chapter, relevant aspects of the law relating to medication for mental health patients are considered. It is beyond the scope of this book to offer a detailed discussion of legal control of mental health care: for this the reader is referred to texts such as Jones, 1991, Williams, 1990 or Montgomery, 1997.

An important consideration when considering some of the legal issues surrounding medication of clients with mental health problems is the extent to which the person is able to make a rational informed decision about his/her treatment. If the illness is such that the client is unable to give informed consent to treatment, then it becomes necessary for health professionals to act in that person's best interest and, in some cases, to act also in the community's best interests. The law in respect of mental health care is constructed in order to meet these needs – to protect the client, the community and also the health professionals involved in the client's care. In the case of a vulnerable client who cannot give informed consent, treatment is considered lawful if, in the opinion of a responsible body of professionals, the actions are in the client's best interests. The terms of the Mental Health Act 1983 create the framework which governs the provision of such care.

Clearly, a dilemma exists if the effects of a client's mental illness pose a threat to either that person or to those in contact with him/her. As will be seen in the various chapters of this book, in many cases medication forms at least part of management of the mental health problems, but difficulties arise if the client is unable to comply with treatment. If a client is detained for treatment under the terms of Part IV of the Mental Health Act 1983, then that person's right to refuse treatment is significantly curtailed. Medication may be given without the individual's consent for 3 months from the date of admission to a mental hospital, following which time the effectiveness of the treatment must be evaluated. If further treatment is needed, but the client remains unwilling to comply, a plan of care including a longer term strategy for medication must be reviewed by the psychiatrist in conjunction with another providing a second opinion. Following this, a report is submitted to the Mental Health Act Commission. As long as the proposed treatment is not irreversible in nature, or otherwise hazardous, emergency measures enable the procedures to be waived in situations in which immediate treatment is needed either to prevent serious deterioration or to save a client's life. In the case of clients whose violent behaviour poses a hazard to self and others, treatment may be given under Sections 57 and 58 of the Mental Health Act as long as the treatment is given in such a way as to provide minimal disruption to the client.

Key point ▶

> The difficulties in giving ethical treatment to clients who are unable to give their informed consent has resulted in the creation of a legal framework to regulate the provision of care.

Medicines and the law

Generally, someone who would benefit from pharmacological treatment must consent to receive medication. When the client gives such consent, s/he is entitled to expect that the drug to be given will be appropriate and as free from adverse effects as possible.

The terms of the Medicines Act 1968 specify the controls under which medicines are produced, advertised, distributed and sold. Before a drug can be offered on the pharmaceutical market, it must be licensed, under the control of the Department of Health. This is the ultimate responsibility of the Secretary of State. Rigorous testing procedures are employed before licensing occurs. The Medicines Act is enforced by a range of bodies, including the Committee on Safety of Medicines.

Once a drug is registered, legislation exists to ensure its safe and appropriate use. Much health care occurs in non-institutional settings and, in law, medication may be administered by the client him/herself or by lay carers. The Medicines Act defines a series of drug categories in order to identify who may have access to the various substances. Some substances are available over-the-counter without the need to consult any authority. The next category of medication may be obtained from a pharmacist with no need for a prescription, and the third category, prescription-only medicine (abbreviated to POM), requires prior consultation with a suitable health professional, usually a medical or dental practitioner, although certain specified preparations may be prescribed by nurses or midwives.

Some drugs have effects that render them susceptible to misuse; in other words, they tend to create physical or mental dependency. The Misuse of Drugs Regulations 1985 further control the availability of these, by subdividing them into five categories, known as schedules.

Schedule 1 drugs are addictive substances that are not used for medicinal purposes. **Schedule 2** encompasses the major stimulants such as the amphetamines and opiate preparations (see Chapter 5). **Schedule 3** comprises barbiturates and minor stimulants (see Chapter 7), **schedule 4** the benzodiazepine tranquillisers (see Chapter 2) and **schedule 5** the controlled drugs that carry only a slight risk of abuse.

Prescriptions

Schedule 2 and 3 drugs are available only by a prescription, which must be written in an indelible medium (usually ink) and signed legibly by the prescriber. The prescription must include the name and address of the client and the dosage to be taken must be specified in both figures and words to minimise the risk of errors occurring. Prescriptions for controlled drugs must be hand-written, specifying the client's name.

Drugs given on a 'named patient' basis

Sometimes, adequate treatment of a client's symptoms is not possible with licensed products and the doctor must resort to preparations that are still being evaluated. Section 9 of the Medicines Act allows regulated use of these products by medical or dental practitioners on a 'named patient' basis. Clients such as pregnant or lactating women or children may need treatment on such a basis because many products are unlicensed for use in these categories of client as insufficient knowledge about their effects is available. In all cases, a reporting mechanism enables prescribers to register any untoward effects that are noted when their client receives pharmaceutical treatment.

Key point ▶

> Because of the inherent ethical difficulties in providing an exhaustive evaluation of safety, only a limited number of drugs are licensed for use in children and pregnant or breastfeeding women.

Information regarding medication

The labelling and marketing of drugs is governed by law. Drug labels must display the name, active substances and form in which the product is presented. In addition, the manufacturer must provide a sheet containing instructions for use, contraindications, warnings and precautions. Drugs supplied for particular patients must be labelled with the recipient's name along with the instructions for use. According to law, information leaflets must be supplied that include the generic name of the product as well as the brand name; the active ingredients, therapeutic uses, contraindications, precautions and common interactions. The latter include effects associated with tobacco, alcohol and food as well as with other drugs. In addition, special warnings must be given related to activities such as driving or operating heavy machinery. The normal dosage, frequency and route of administration must also be specified, along with instructions in case of overdosage and any known withdrawal effects.

It is against the law to advertise prescription drugs to the public.

Key point ▶

> The amount of information available to the client about a pharmaceutical product is specified by law.

Storage of drugs

Schedules 1, 2 and 3 'controlled' drugs are subject to regulations related to their storage: they must be stored in a locked cupboard within another locked cupboard and a warning light must be fitted to indicate when the cupboard is open. The administration of drugs categorised within schedule 2 must be recorded within a bound register in which the name of each recipient is recorded, in addition to the formulation of the substance, the amount given and the remaining balance.

Key point ▶

> Drugs are subject to rigorous testing prior to being licensed for use. During this process, the preparation is classified according to its potential for misuse, and this governs its overall availability and control related to storage and administration.

SUMMARY

In this chapter, we have considered the principles by which cells communicate, and how these mechanisms are organised within the central nervous system. Subsequently, some of the principles of pharmacology were reviewed, including the legal controls that govern and restrict drug usage so as to protect the client, society and, in some cases, the health professionals themselves.

REFERENCES AND FURTHER READING

Carlson, N.R. (2001) *Physiology of Behaviour*, 7th edn. Allyn & Bacon, Boston.

Johnson, D.L., Wiebe, J.S., Gold, S.M. *et al.* (1999) Cerebral blood flow and personality: a positron emission tomography study. *American Journal of Psychiatry*, **156**, 252–257.

Jones, R. (1991) *Mental Health Act Manual*. Sweet & Maxwell, London.

Montgomery, J. (1997) *Health Care Law*. Oxford University Press, Oxford.

Sacks, O. (1995) *An Anthropologist on Mars*. Picador, London.

Williams, J. (1990) *The Law of Mental Health*. Fourmat Publishing, London.

Yager, J., Siegfried, S.L. and DiMatteo, T.L. (1999) Use of alternative remedies by psychiatric patients: illustrative vignettes and a discussion of the issues. *American Journal of Psychiatry*, **156**, 1432–1438.

Website

Drug poisoning: http://factmonster.com/ce6/sci/A0816136.html

SELF-TEST QUESTIONS

Identify which of the following options are likely to apply. Some, all or none of the statements may be correct.

1. The characteristic that distinguishes a nerve cell from others is that it:
   a. communicates with other tissues
   b. has the quality of irritability
   c. can pump ions into its cytoplasm via ion channels to alter polarity
   d. releases hormones as a result of stimulation
2. Which of the following statements are true?
   a. the nervous system is the rapid communication system within the body
   b. the endocrine system is regulated by a system of feedback mechanisms
   c. cells can regulate the number of endocrine receptors according to hormone levels
   d. the endocrine system communicates more slowly than the nervous system
3. When considering administering a drug to a client, the nurse

should remember that:

a.   the addition of another drug to a medication regime may alter bioavailability

b.   medication given by mouth is absorbed more rapidly than that given parenterally

c.   the formulation of depot injections delays transport of the drug to the target tissues

d.   toxicity may occur if hepatic or renal impairment is present

4.   A client needs medication for a mental health problem. Substances given to act upon the brain must be able to:

a.   influence the endocrine system

b.   cross the blood/brain barrier

c.   act as a neurotransmitter

d.   be rapidly excreted

5.   Because of the mechanics of first-pass metabolism:

a.   it is inadvisable to mix drugs with alcohol

b.   medication is sometimes administered parenterally

c.   the client should maintain an adequate fluid intake

d.   oral doses tend to be larger than those for parenteral administration.

6.   Which of these statements about drug excretion are correct?

a.   in stage 1 metabolism some molecules of the drug remain pharmacologically active

b.   in stage 1 metabolism, the drug molecules become water-soluble

c.   in stage 2 metabolism the drug molecules have become pharmacologically inactive;

d.   in stage 2 metabolism the drug molecules have become water soluble

7.   A client commences a prescription for a mental health problem. The health professional should be aware that:

a.   the client should be encouraged to read the information leaflet supplied

b.   the prescriber should have been informed of other medication in use

c.   the medication will not become effective until therapeutic levels in the CNS are achieved

d.   if taken concurrently, herbal preparations may interact with the pharmaceutical preparation

8.   Therapeutic levels of a drug are influenced by:

a.   the levels of plasma protein

b.   the client's compliance with treatment

c.   whether or not the client smokes cigarettes

d.   the choice of route for administration

9.   A client may be given compulsory medication if:

a.   the treatment is not irreversible in nature

b.   Part IV of the Mental Health Act (1983) is invoked

c.   the drug is licensed by the Committee of Safety of Medicines

d.   the drug is a prescription-only medicine
10.   Which of these drugs fall within Schedule 4 of the Misuse of Drugs Regulations 1985?
   a.   cannabis
   b.   amphetamines
   c.   barbiturates
   d.   benzodiazepines

2 ALTERED AROUSAL: ANXIETY AND ANXIETY-RELATED DISORDERS

INTRODUCTION

This chapter will discuss the normal bodily response to challenging situations and the disorders that ensue when there is a mismatch between challenge and the mental and physiological response to it. Drugs used in the treatment of anxiety states will be indicated as appropriate within sections discussing the various mechanisms that govern anxiety. The products commonly used at present will be discussed in further detail in the section headed 'Drugs used in the treatment of anxiety'. An anxious person commonly has alterations to the normal sleeping patters so sleep disorders will be discussed in the last part of the chapter.

Anxiety disorders can be explained using a range of approaches using psychodynamic, psychoanalytic, behavioural, cognitive, genetic and biological theories. As this book is primarily about psychopharmacological treatment, it is the biological theories that will be considered here.

EFFECTS OF THREATENING STIMULI UPON CEREBRAL FUNCTION

The arousal response involves an interaction between the neural and endocrine systems. As creatures evolved and began to live more interesting lives than simply ingesting and metabolising nutrients and replicating themselves, it became important to be able to recognise danger and to mount responses to deal with threatening situations. This required internal communication mechanisms to coordinate appropriate mental and physical functioning.

In order for a danger to be registered, the brain must enter a state of arousal. Various neurotransmitter systems are involved in the creation of cerebral arousal. These include serotonin (5-hydroxytryptamine, 5-HT), noradrenaline (norepinephrine), dopamine, adenosine and the benzodiazepine/gamma-aminobutyric acid (GABA) receptor systems (Cates *et al.*, 1996). The noradrenergic neurones are predominantly located within the brain stem in the locus ceruleus. This structure has neural projections linking it to the limbic system, cerebral cortex and the cerebellum. The locus ceruleus is activated if threatening situations are encountered. Normally, the effect of the transmitters producing arousal is in balance with the effect of transmitters, such as GABA, that inhibit arousal. The interaction between these transmitter systems

Key point ▶

> Normally a balance exists between the mechanisms that produce neural excitation and suppression. In such cases, anxiety levels remain within normal limits.

mediates normal and maladaptive anxiety responses. Should this balance be lost, anxiety may become disabling.

The arousal response: integration of neural and endocrine responses

There are two major systems that provide internal communication mechanisms. The fastest and most obvious system involves neural responses within the central, peripheral and autonomic nervous systems. Neural responses require effector systems to carry out the orders from the brain. Implementation and potentiation of neural commands takes place as a result of endocrine responses, which prepare systems for 'fright, fight or flight' by releasing muscle fuels from store, speeding cellular metabolism to cope with the increased level of demand and preparing the body to deal with possible injury.

As animals evolved, the arousal mechanism was created to deal with physical challenge, such as the risk of becoming another creature's meal or having to compete for food or a mate. Our response to stress is therefore to some extent an evolutionary throwback: when we get 'butterflies' before an examination or important interview, or when the computer crashes with a precious piece of work inside it, we have to harness responses that were originally designed to enable us to run away from the danger or to fight an aggressor. Although we may wish to be able to deal with the examination or interview by removing ourselves rapidly from the scene, or respond to the infuriating computer by attacking it with a hammer, modern-day difficulties are usually made worse instead of better by the use of such tactics. The result is that, in certain circumstances, we may become unwell because we are using relatively obsolete mechanisms to cope with present-day challenges. It may also help to explain why some people 'run away' mentally from a challenging situation, even though they may remain physically present.

The acute response to challenge

It is interesting that the lay language used to describe an acute challenge acknowledges the underlying physiological mechanisms, even though the speaker may not understand them in any detail. A footballer being interviewed after a successful match will often refer to 'the adrenaline flowing' or being 'pumped up'. People experiencing emotional trauma may refer to 'an icy hand' clutching 'the stomach', or to a situation 'making their hair stand on end'. Stress can be described as the body's response to a demand. Most people perceive stress as an uncomfortable and possibly dangerous experience.

However, it is interesting to consider the impact of challenge upon everyday performance. People often seek a change of employment because they feel that their existing lifestyle is insufficiently challenging. Health-care workers and other people whose work intensity can fluctuate are not always pleased when the demands of work drop below a certain level as they may find that the time goes slowly and they feel disinclined to do what work there is to be done. Conversely, and

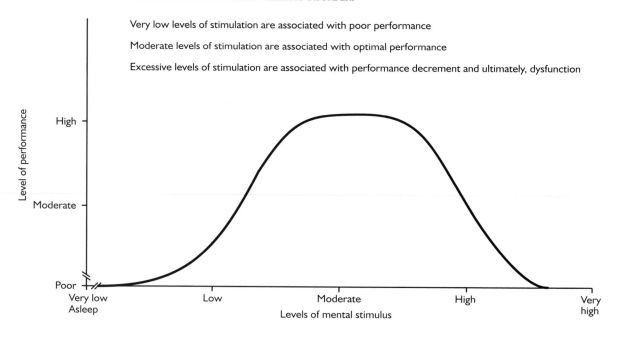

Very low levels of stimulation are associated with poor performance

Moderate levels of stimulation are associated with optimal performance

Excessive levels of stimulation are associated with performance decrement and ultimately, dysfunction

Figure 2.1

Stress and performance: the inverted U-shaped curve

perhaps more commonly in today's health-care arena, when the work intensity increases above a certain threshold, effectiveness diminishes and the person begins to suffer excessive fatigue, emotional blunting and increased incidence of minor illnesses. These may be the warning signs of 'burnout'. This relationship between levels of arousal and quality of performance was originally examined by Yerkes and Dodson (1908) and may be plotted as an inverted-U-shaped curve (Figure 2.1). At a certain level of arousal, performance is optimal and the individual enjoys the feeling of being effective. At the physiological level, the systemic responses and the challenge are matched, and the result is mood and performance enhancement.

The acute response to challenge may be demonstrated by the example of an athlete in the final moments before a race. The person feels 'keyed up', may have an inability to keep still, feel tense and experience tremor, palpitations and an increased rate of breathing. The same feelings are experienced by the person waiting to enter the examination hall. The night before the examination there may have been sleep disturbance and while waiting to begin the examination there may be feelings of nausea and the skin may become sweaty. This response was described by Hans Selye (1976) as the general adaptation syndrome, a classical explanation of the response to short-term and sustained challenge. Selye described three stages: stage 1, the 'alarm reaction', in which preparation is made for 'fright, fight or fight'; stage 2, 'resistance', which deals with longer-term stressors; and stage 3, which is a dysfunctional 'exhaustion' stage in which illness or death may result from the effects of sustained psychological challenge.

Box 2.1

'Feel good' molecules

Those who engage in regular exercise of reasonably high intensity will recognise the sense of wellbeing after a challenging workout or race. At such times the physical body is experienced as an efficiently running machine, and negative moods and pain are suppressed and lost as the individual is immersed in the physical activity. It is only when the marathon runner crosses the finish line that s/he may collapse or notice pain as a result of the sustained physical demand. This moderation of the sensory apparatus is thought to occur as a result of release of peptides (short chains of amino acids), which inhibit transmission of pain impulses between the sensory nerve endings and the cerebral cortex. These molecules were first identified in the 1970s and were linked with a large range of physiological responses but were especially associated with the euphoria and reduction of pain perception that working athletes experience. They were named endorphins and enkephalins and were demonstrated to bind with naturally occurring receptors to which opiate analgesics such as morphine attached. In the chapter discussing depression, the importance of neurotransmitter substances in the control of normal mood is explained. Endorphins, as well as altering the pain response, produce a sense of peace and may be considered as naturally occurring tranquillisers!

The arousal response that generates feelings of anxiety was originally a safety mechanism that enabled a rapid response to threatening stimuli.

The acute stress response enables the person to respond to the alarm reaction. The rapid response system is the sympathetic nervous system in association with the central nervous system (CNS) where interpretation and reasoning occur and the peripheral nervous system where communication is made with effector structures such as muscles and joints in readiness to move the person or animal away from danger. The startle response is seen better in animals such as deer or horses than in humans, who have evolved away from exploiting their less impressive skill in running away from danger, even although the original stress mechanisms remain.

As can be seen in Figure 2.2, the sympathetic mechanisms prepare the body for an intensive physical effort in order to move the individual away from trouble fast. The sympathetic system is designed for instant reaction and its effects are boosted by secretions from the adrenal medulla. The sympathetic nerves innervate the adrenal medulla stimulating the release of adrenaline (epinephrine) and noradrenaline (norepinephrine), enhancing the sympathetic response. In the CNS, noradrenaline is a neurotransmitter that helps to govern mood (Figure 2.3; see above and Chapter 3)

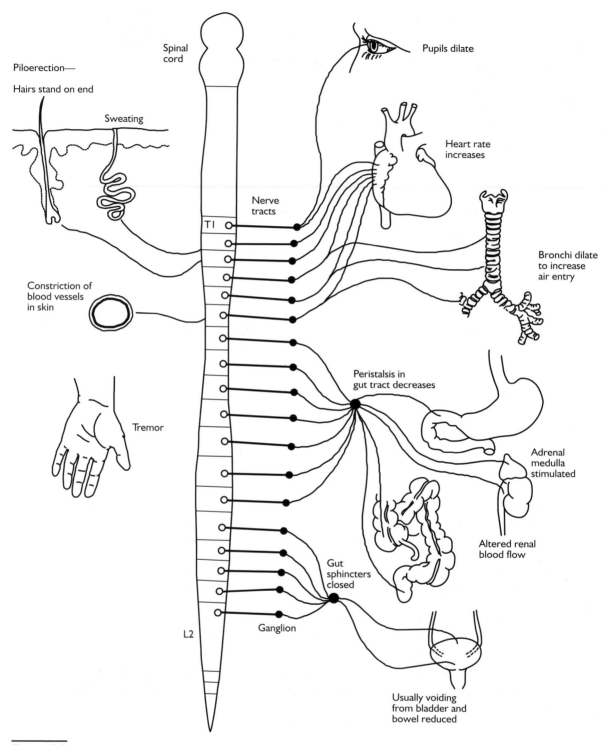

Figure 2.2

Short-term arousal: effects of sympathetic nervous system stimulation

The acute alarm response: Effects of adrenaline and noradrenaline

ADRENALINE

Dilatation of pupils - distance vision enhanced
Cutaneous vasoconstriction
Constriction of gut blood vessels
Relaxation of gut muscles
Constriction of gut sphincters
Responsiveness of bladder wall reduced
Constriction of bladder sphincters

Stimulation of cardiac muscle producing increased rate and force of contraction

Bronchodilation
Respiratory rate increased

Increased skeletal muscle tone

Mobilisation of stored glycogen and fats
Increased metabolic rate

Increased coagulability of blood

Contraction of arrectores pylii in skin

NORADRENALINE
Generalised peripheral vasoconstriction
Elevation of blood pressure

The effects of sympathetic nervous system stimulation are therefore enhanced

The body is prepared to respond to emergencies and threatening situations

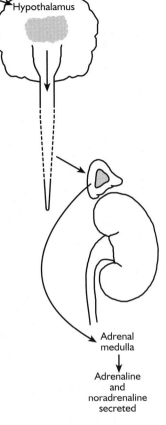

Anxiety
Hypothalamus

Adrenal medulla

Adrenaline and noradrenaline secreted

Figure 2.3

Short-term arousal: effects of adrenal stimulation

'Good' stress

Adrenaline secretion is associated with a sense of satisfaction as a result of meeting a challenge. This may go some way towards explaining why some people seek out challenges, whether they involve bungee jumping, seeking a demanding job in an acute admissions unit or waiting until the last minute before writing an assignment for college. The response to stress seems to work best when the nature of the challenge is unambiguous and when the increased effort takes place over a comparatively short time and is drawn to a clear, preferably positive, conclusion. Such 'healthy' stress is known as **eustress**.

> A certain amount of neural arousal is important to ensure optimal performance

◄ **Key point**

Maladaptive stress

It can be seen that the stress response is often beneficial and may in fact be actively sought by some people. If a person had no ability to respond to acute physiological changes within the body, then death might occur, as in the case of people with Addison's disease, whose adrenal glands fail and who are unable to maintain their blood pressure and cardiac function should they become acutely ill. Some forms of stress, however, have been associated with distress and illness. Long-term stress, often associated with an uncertain outcome, involves different physiological mechanisms from the acute stress response. When a person becomes distressed, a sustained response is needed. Effort is made without the reward of satisfaction: all that is experienced is a sense of continuing demand, usually raising the question of whether the individual can meet that demand.

Longer term responses to challenge

Distress is the result of a sense of threat rather than an achievable challenge. While the challenge mechanism involves the cerebral cortex, sympathetic nervous system and the secretions of the adrenal medulla, distress involves an emotional response via the limbic system, activation of the hypothalamus and pituitary gland, release of adrenocorticotrophic hormone and subsequent release of cortisol (hydrocortisone)

Figure 2.4

Effects of sustained response to perceived threat

Effects of aldosterone

Sodium and water conservation
Increased potassium loss via urine
Increased hydrogen ion loss via urine

Effects of cortisol

Increased glucose production
Increased protein and fat breakdown
Suppression of immune system

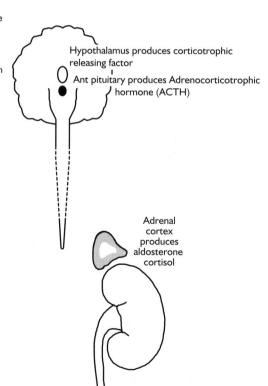

Hypothalamus produces corticotrophic releasing factor

Ant pituitary produces Adrenocorticotrophic hormone (ACTH)

Adrenal cortex produces aldosterone cortisol

and aldosterone (Figure 2.4). For further explanation of some of the physical effects of sustained threat, see Chapter 8.

ANXIETY DISORDERS AND THE MANNER IN WHICH ANXIOLYTIC DRUGS PRINCIPALLY WORK

Anxiety disorders were discussed by Hippocrates in the 4th century BC but were not considered to have any significant effect upon health until approximately 30 years ago (Mendlowicz and Stein, 2000). Anxiety disorders include general anxiety disorders, social phobia and specific phobias, panic disorders with or without agoraphobia, post-traumatic stress disorder (PTSD) and obsessive–compulsive disorder (OCD). Mendlowicz and Stein (2000) conducted a review of studies examining the impact of anxiety disorders upon quality of life and concluded that most anxiety disorders cause significant impairment of quality of life and social interaction.

> Anxiety disorders are a common source of reduced quality of life.

◄ **Key point**

Many anxiolytic preparations take their effect by decreasing the rate of neuronal firing within the locus ceruleus. Corticotrophic releasing factor is secreted within the locus ceruleus and its production is reduced by the drug **alprazolam**. Corticotrophic releasing factor is thought to be responsible for coordinating the behavioural, neural and endocrine responses to a stressful situation. In post-traumatic stress disorder, cortisol levels have been found to be depleted (Cates *et al.*, 1996). Caffeine, which can increase subjective anxiety, increases the activity of the locus ceruleus. This stimulatory effect is balanced by the inhibitory transmitter GABA, which binds to $GABA_A$ and $GABA_B$ receptors. Benzodiazepines bind to $GABA_A$ receptors, changing the shape of these, and increase the affinity of GABA, thus increasing the rate of binding at these sites. As a result, neural transmission is suppressed and subjective anxiety is reduced.

> The anxiety response is mediated within the locus ceruleus where corticotrophic releasing factor is secreted to fuel the anxiety response.

◄ **Key point**

The mechanism by which GABA is produced and released

Gamma-aminobutyric acid, a 'calming' transmitter, is made from intraneural stores of the amino acid precursor glutamate as a result of the action of the enzyme glutamic acid decarboxylase. Glutamate is present in abundance within the CNS. When the relevant neurones are stimulated, GABA is released at the presynaptic nerve endings into the synapse. It is subsequently taken back into the presynaptic cleft for storage until further use is required. GABA is broken down by the enzyme GABA transaminase ($GABA_t$). Two types of receptor, $GABA_A$ and $GABA_B$, regulate nerve transmission and this process is also influenced by an assortment of other local receptors, such as the benzodiazepine and anticonvulsant receptors. Nerve function in anxiety is thus controlled by a multiplicity of factors and molecules within the CNS. It is generally thought that it is only the $GABA_A$ receptors that are involved in the mechanism of anxiety (Stahl, 1996).

Benzodiazepine receptors

Researchers became aware of the presence of benzodiazepine receptors when examining the action of the benzodiazepine tranquillisers. During this process, they noted that the molecules of tranquilliser became bound to neural structures that appeared to be 'purpose built' for them. It appears that there are three types of benzodiazepine receptor. Benzodiazepine-1 receptors are particularly present in the cerebellum. The pharmacological actions influencing anxiety reduction and promotion of sleep seem to work mainly through the benzodiazepine-1 receptor system. Benzodiazepine-2 receptors are mainly found within the spinal cord and corpus striatum and are involved with muscle relaxation. Benzodiazepine-3 receptors are found within the kidney and at present their purpose is unclear (Figure 2.5).

Drugs taking effect in the locality of the benzodiazepine receptors tend to reduce anxiety, relax muscle, promote sleep or control convulsive seizures. It is thought that activity at these sites may also influence drug dependency and withdrawal mechanisms. It is likely that there are natural substances that exert the same effects, although these remain at present largely undiscovered.

Key point ▶

> The presence of receptors that accept benzodiazepine drugs suggests that naturally occurring molecules may be produced to generate tranquillity.

The $GABA_A$ and benzodiazepine receptor mechanisms respectively work in synchrony to control the movement of chloride ions via channels in the neural membrane. When the two receptor systems work in synchrony, movement of chlorides into the nerve is greatly increased, and neural transmission is reduced (Figure 2.5). Thus, joint activity between the $GABA_A$ and benzodiazepine receptors reduces the generation of action potentials, suppresses neural activity and diminishes the subjective sensation of anxiety.

(a) Normal stimulation results in ion channels allowing passage of positively charged ions into neurone to create an action potential

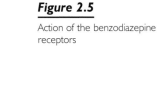

Figure 2.5

Action of the benzodiazepine receptors

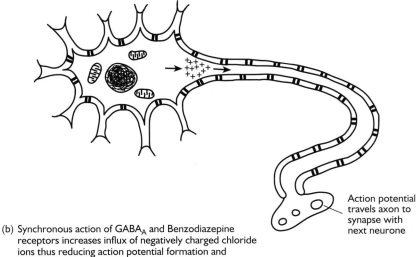

Action potential travels axon to synapse with next neurone

(b) Synchronous action of GABA$_A$ and Benzodiazepine receptors increases influx of negatively charged chloride ions thus reducing action potential formation and quietening nerve activity

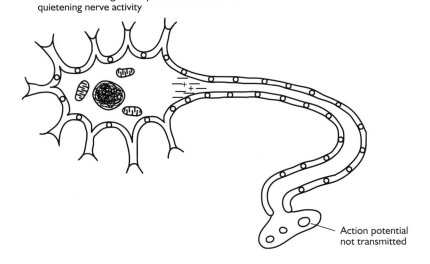

Action potential not transmitted

CASE STUDY 2.1   JESS, A CLIENT WITH ANXIETY

Read this case study and then, when you have read the sections on anxiety and its treatment, attempt to answer the questions that follow.

Jess is your next-door neighbour and she knows you work in mental health. For some time, she has been bothered by feelings of anxiety. Often she can find no real cause for this, just a general feeling of unease. The problem has been getting worse over the past year. Now her weekends are often spoiled because, by Sunday morning, she has begun to worry about returning to work on Monday. Sometimes, when she thinks about work, her intestines seem to give a sharp twist and she feels nauseous. When she goes to bed at night, her mind seems to go into overdrive, so she has difficulty sleeping. Her worries are exhausting, and her abdominal problems mean that she rarely feels like eating a proper meal. She decides that she had better visit her family doctor to get some help as her life is becoming ever more uncomfortable.

Jess is prescribed gepirone and is advised that it might be a while before she really begins to feel better. Having left the surgery, she wonders why she couldn't have been given something to take the anxious feelings away quickly.

Jess asks you whether she can take alcohol, as she cannot remember what the doctor told her – she was too anxious at the time!

1. What might Jess's doctor have given her that would have been faster acting? Why do you think s/he did not do so?
2. Can Jess take alcohol with gepirone? What would you say in answer to her question?

CASE STUDY 2.2   FERGAL, A CLIENT WITH SOCIAL PHOBIA

Read this case study and then, when you have read the sections on anxiety and social phobia, attempt to answer the questions that follow.

Fergal is a 32-year-old man who develops computer software for a living. He knows he is clever with computers but feels he is very stupid as far as other people are concerned. He is absolutely fine with the computers, as they don't have expectations of him, and he is happy to do overtime working on problems. This has, for him, the happy effect that he is much too busy to go to any social functions. The problem is that he has become more and more reluctant to speak to people: even standing at the supermarket checkout has become an ordeal as people always seem to want to make conversation. Now, however, he fears he is ill, as he has palpitations and feels jittery. He hates handing over change in shops as he suspects that the shop assistants are disgusted by the money, which is damp from his sweaty hands. Finally he plucks up courage to seek help and finds to his surprise that he has been prescribed drugs that he knows are antidepressants. He has also been referred for some specialist treatment.

1. What sort of antidepressants is he likely to have been prescribed?.
2. What sort of therapy might also help him?

As can be seen in Box 2.2, the action of the benzodiazepine receptors can be influenced by drugs that increase the movement of chlorides (benzodiazepine agonists) or by those that decrease the movement of chlorides along the ion channels into the nerve (benzodiazepine antagonists).

Box 2.2

Clinical effect of modification of the chloride ion channels

- **Benzodiazepine agonists** increase the movement of chlorides into the nerve, producing an inhibition of neural transmission and as a result reducing anxiety and tendency to convulsive seizures and decreasing memory formation
- **Inverse benzodiazepine agonists** decrease the movement of chloride ions, promote anxiety, increase tendency to convulsions and increase memory formation

- **Partial agonists** can be useful for maximising the desired effect (anxiety reduction) while minimising undesired effects (daytime sleepiness, ataxia, memory impairment, emotional withdrawal and benzodiazepine dependency)
- **The benzodiazepine antagonist flumazenil** blocks the action of the benzodiazepines and reverses their effect, which is useful in the treatment of overdosage

Excess of serotonin at post synaptic receptors are thought to cause shutting down (down regulation) of serotonin I_A receptors

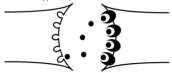 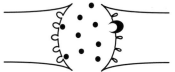

Figure 2.6

Interaction between the GABA$_A$ and benzodiazepine receptor mechanisms and the effect upon nerve transmission

- Serotonin is taken up more slowly, increased concentration in the synapses results → increased rate of transmission → sensations of anxiety.

Normally, a balance is maintained between the amount of free serotonin and the number of available receptors.

Medication

◊ Serotonin I_A (5 H-TI_A) partial agonists, e.g. gepirone; tandospirone; ipsapirone; venlafaxine XR.

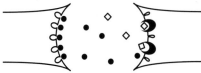

compete for receptors. When bound to these, a less powerful effect is obtained than would be the case if serotonin was in situ. Thus, transmission is reduced, anxiety is gradually brought under control without producing excessive sedation or exacerbating existing depression.

Benzodiazepines

Benzodiazepine tranquillizers bind to GABA$_A$ and GABA$_B$ receptors, changing their shape and thus allowing more GABA to bind, reducing the rate of neurone transmission and producing a calming effect. These drugs are therefore receptor agonists.

 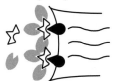

Anxiety and the noradrenaline transmitter system

Most noradrenaline-secreting neurones are positioned with their nerve cell body in the locus ceruleus in the brain stem. Overactivity of these noradrenergic neurones is thought to contribute to anxiety states. The nerve cell bodies of the locus ceruleus and presynaptic nerve terminals throughout the brain have alpha-2 noradrenaline receptors. A feedback mechanism is thought to exist in which the nerve cell bodies in the locus ceruleus and the alpha-2 receptors regulate the amount of noradrenaline released by the nerve endings. If the mechanism is inhibited by receptor blocking agents, the overall output of noradrenaline is increased, locus ceruleus activity is greater and anxiety is experienced. If the receptors are bound to alpha-1 agonist agents, then the overall effect is a reduction of subjective anxiety. **Clonidine** is such a noradrenergic blocker that is used in this way as an anxiolytic medication.

Noradrenaline bound to beta-adrenergic receptors produces sensations of anxiety. The combination increases the rate of neuronal firing in the locus ceruleus nerves and generates the experience of anxiety. When noradrenergic neurones are excessively stimulated, superfluous noradrenaline is released in the vicinity of the receptors, particularly the beta-adrenergic receptors, and the anxiety response is enhanced. Administration of beta-blockers such as **propranolol** will produce an anxiolytic effect.

The serotonin theory of anxiety generation

A simple view of this is that excessive serotonin at the nerve endings will evoke anxiety while depletion will result in depression. Manipulation of the serotonin levels within the synapse should improve depressive states, as is explained in Chapter 3. Some clients suffer from depression with anxiety, which would not be effectively treated with straightforward selective serotonin receptor inhibitor (SSRI) preparations. Products have now been developed that act as partial serotonin agonists. These work by modulating serotonin levels so as to partially improve the depression while avoiding the increased neuronal activity that would cause anxiety and agitation. Preparations affecting the serotonin-1A (5-HT1A) receptors show promise in the treatment of anxiety that complicates depression.

Key point ▶

> Increased levels of serotonin at certain synapses will contribute to an overall increase in feelings of anxiety.

It is thought that, in anxiety states, a persistent excess of serotonin at the synapses may cause the serotonin-1A receptors to downregulate (reduce) their sensitivity, as opposed to the situation in depression, in which the receptors may upregulate (increase) their sensitivity because of a depletion of the neurotransmitter. (For an overview of this process of regulation of the number and sensitivity of cell membrane receptors, see the sections on cellular communication in Chapter 1.) It is thought that there may be families of serotonin receptor subtypes and that serotonin-1A receptor activity may have a role in mediating the anxiety response. Serotonin-1A partial agonists may act upon serotonin receptors, helping neurones to re-balance the altered serotonin levels and the response of the serotonin receptors. Serotonin-1A partial agonists are thought to slow the adaptations made by the receptors and thus to produce a delayed response and a slow anxiolytic effect, as opposed to the rapid anxiolytic response which is achieved through activation of the benzodiazepine receptors. Examples of serotonin-1A partial agonists include the **buspirone**-related compounds, for example **gepirone**, **tandospirone** and **ipsapirone**.

◀ **Key point**

> Mood levels are probably balanced normally by synaptic receptors regulating neural susceptibility to serotonin. This same mechanism is manipulated by serotonin-1A partial agonist drugs, which enable gradual correction of excessive anxiety.

Figure 2.6 shows how the partial agonist competes with serotonin for binding sites at the serotonin-1A receptors. The partial agonist is less powerful in effect than natural serotonin. At first, there is no noticeable effect, then, gradually, anxiety diminishes as the neurone's overall response to the stimulating effect of serotonin decreases. Figure 2.7 summarises the mechanisms which are currently thought to contribute to the development of anxiety disorders.

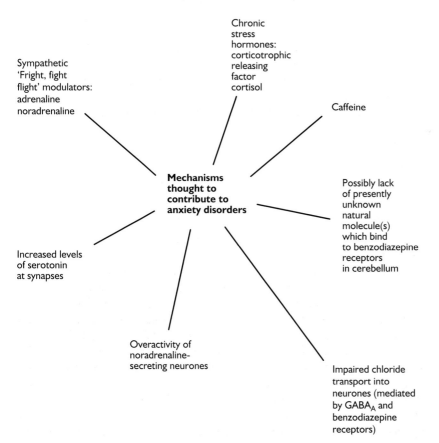

Figure 2.7

Mechanisms possibly contributing to the development of anxiety

Understanding the anxious patient

Anxiety as a result of a stressor is a normal response, termed **situational anxiety** and usually lasting no more than a few weeks. The patient may find a mild anxiolytic agent beneficial. Anxiety may accompany mental illnesses such as depression, dementia, schizophrenia, mania or substance misuse. Some stimulant substances, such as amphetamines, isoprenaline, nicotine, caffeine and the nasal decongestant ephedrine evoke feelings of anxiety. Early attempts at pharmacological treatment of anxiety simply involved sedation to relieve the physical symptoms associated with anxiety and thus acted purely to mask the condition while substituting the problems of sedation for the original anxiety.

Key point ▶

> Selection of appropriate treatment of anxiety disorders depends upon the severity and duration of the anxiety and whether or not the client also has depression.

General anxiety disorder

Sufferers from this disabling form of anxiety experience untoward worry that is difficult to control and that lasts for 6 months or more. The anxiety is associated with three or more of the following symptoms: fatigue, problems with concentration, irritability, restlessness, disturbed sleep and muscular tension. The patient may have stress-related physical symptoms such as headache or irritable bowel disease and also feel depressed. Epidemiological studies have indicated that general anxiety disorder occurs more frequently in people who are unmarried or divorced, and its overall effects upon the client's lifestyle are considered to be as disabling as those of depression. Females are more frequently affected than males and general anxiety disorder (GAD) is more common when there is a family history of anxiety and depression. GAD may first present when the client is in his/her twenties and last for 20 years, and rarely remits spontaneously (Rickels *et al.*, 2000). It carries a 20% chance of recovery. The long-standing presence of this condition is associated with the development of panic disorder (see below).

Sufferers from GAD may be helped by the prescription of short-term benzodiazepine anxiolytics to enable control of sudden increases in their symptoms and to stabilise their state in the short term, but adjunctive techniques such as stress reduction activities and lifestyle management support become an important part of their care, although discussion of these is beyond the scope of this book.

Because of the nature of this disorder, sufferers from GAD often require long-standing medication. **Lorazepam**, a benzodiazepine, and **buspirone** are used to treat the condition, as are tricyclic antidepressants such as **imipramine**, which has been found to be effective in GAD that is accompanied by major depression. Selective serotonin reuptake inhibitors; and antidepressants such as **trazodone** and **nefazodone** are also used to treat this condition.

◀ **Key point**

> General anxiety disorders require treatment that may be continued over a protracted length of time.

The use of extended-release venlafaxine **(venlafaxine XR)**, an antidepressant that is chemically similar to imipramine, has been evaluated as useful in a controlled trial in non-depressed sufferers from GAD in the USA (Rickels *et al.*, 2000). Venlafaxine acts upon the serotonin and noradrenaline systems and has been found to be an effective anxiolytic without the adverse reactions associated with the benzodiazepines. The relative lack of side-effects make it tolerable for the client to take, although occasionally nausea, insomnia and dizziness have been experienced. Other side-effects that have been noted are dryness of the mouth, sleepiness and generalised weakness. Withdrawal symptoms sometimes occur when the treatment is ceased or tapered off. These include fatigue, headache, nausea and vomiting, dizziness, dry mouth, diarrhoea, insomnia, feelings of nervousness, sweating, vertigo and paraesthesia ('pins and needles').

In overdose, venlafaxine may cause alterations to the pulse rate, either tachycardias or bradycardias, and seizures may occur, although these effects are rare and usually self-limiting. There is no particular antidote: activated charcoal may be given and the pulse and blood pressure should be watched closely.

Examples of benzodiazepines used to treat clients with generalised anxiety disorder include **alprazolam** to a maximum dose of 1 mg four times daily, **chlordiazepoxide, clonazepam, chlorazepate, diazepam, halazepam** and **lorazepam**. Results of a study evaluating the effects of lorazepam on two groups of subjects with high and low levels of anxiety respectively suggest that benzodiazepines may exert different effects depending upon the client's prevailing level of arousal (Garcia *et al.*, 2000). Benzodiazepines such as diazepam and clorazepate combine readily with lipids, making them able to enter the CNS readily and thus provide rapid relief from anxiety. This provides the sensation of a 'rush' for some clients, which predisposes to a risk of misuse of these agents.

Pharmacological research continues to develop anxiolytics that offer acceptable treatment for those with long-term GAD.

◀ **Key point**

> Sedative agents such as benzodiazepines, which combine readily with lipids, can produce dramatic improvement in mood. However, this can tempt a client to misuse the drug to obtain mood elevation.

DRUGS USED IN THE TREATMENT OF ANXIETY

Short-term anxiety disorders such as the response to a sudden upsetting life event can be treated for a few weeks or months with benzodiazepine anxiolytics. Clients with long-term conditions such as generalised anxiety disorder or panic disorder are more difficult to help, as long-term benzodiazepine treatment is complicated by dependency symptoms and, later, withdrawal effects when the therapy is finally discontinued.

Buspirone

This product is used for short-term treatment of anxiety disorders. The usual therapeutic dose is 15–30 mg daily in divided doses. The maximum daily total dose is 45 mg, given in divided doses. The dose is built up over a period of days to achieve control of the client's symptoms. Buspirone is unsuitable for clients with epilepsy and care is needed if the client has impaired liver or kidney function. Vigilance and intellectual function is usually unimpaired and the effect is not potentiated by alcohol. Concurrent use with monoamine oxidase inhibitors (MAOIs) is not advised, as hypertension may result.

Buspirone is generally not advised for use during pregnancy and lactation but otherwise appears to be well tolerated. Side-effects are rare but include, dizziness, headaches, nervousness, light-headedness, nausea and excitement. In general, buspirone is relatively safe in overdose, although this situation becomes more complicated if multiple substances have been ingested. The stomach should be emptied and support should be available to ensure adequate cardiovascular and respiratory function.

Nefazodone

Nefazodone may be used for anxiety associated with depression or for sleep disturbances. The normal therapeutic dose is 200 mg twice daily, with a maximum dose of 300 mg twice daily. This dose is built up after about a week of initial treatment. The therapeutic effects build up slowly, so treatment may need to be continued for a period of months. Older female clients may have a tendency to accumulate toxic plasma levels, so they may be prescribed a lower maintenance dose. Adverse effects include weakness, dryness of the mouth, nausea, constipation, lightheadedness, dizziness and sleepiness. Care must be taken if the agent is prescribed for epileptic clients as seizures may be exacerbated. In overdose, the effects of nefazodone are mainly drowsiness and vomiting and the patient may become hypotensive.

Propranolol

Propranolol exerts an anxiolytic effect by blocking the beta-adrenoreceptors of the sympathetic nervous system, thus diminishing the 'fright, fight or flight' response. A long-acting preparation is available. This preparation is useful for controlling situational anxiety and generalised anxiety states. Generally, the product is well tolerated. For anxiety disorders, 80 mg of sustained-release propranolol is usually helpful.

Adverse effects of propranolol include decreased exercise tolerance, fatigue, and cold extremities. Confusion, nightmares, sleep disturbances, psychoses and hallucinations may also occur. Propranolol must not be given to people subject to bronchial asthma, as its action as a sympathetic antagonist will provoke bronchospasm. In overdose, propranolol causes hypotension, bradycardia, shock and bronchospasm.

Trazodone

Trazodone is an antidepressant agent that also has anxiolytic properties. It is a serotonin reuptake inhibitor. The dose for the treatment of anxiety is 75 mg daily, which can be increased to a maximum of 300 mg daily to control the symptoms of anxiety. As it may cause sedation, clients must be warned of the hazard of driving and operating heavy machinery during the first few days of taking this medication. However, the sedative effect diminishes as the treatment continues. Trazodone may produce cardiac rhythm disturbances in susceptible people. In overdosage, it produces drowsiness, dizziness and vomiting.

The benzodiazepines

Alprazolam

Alprazolam is used for short-term treatment of moderate or severe anxiety states and anxiety accompanying depression. The manufacturers recommend that care is taken to avoid long-term treatment because of the problems with benzodiazepine dependence, and that the client is reassessed after 4 weeks to establish whether continuing treatment is necessary. The dose is determined by the extent of the patient's symptoms and the responsiveness to the drug – the aim is to give the lowest dose possible that will control the anxiety. The normal dose range for the treatment of anxiety is between 0.25 mg and 0.5 mg three times daily. The maximum total daily dose is 3 mg. Older clients tend to be more sensitive to alprazolam as they have reduced ability to excrete it. Sedation may impair the client's vigilance, so motoring or operating heavy machinery may be hazardous and the sedative effect is potentiated by alcohol. If alprazolam is needed during the late stages of pregnancy, the newborn baby is likely to suffer hypothermia, respiratory depression and general 'floppiness' due to reduced muscle tone. Box 2.3 lists the signs of dependency and withdrawal.

| Mild symptoms | Anxiety, insomnia, irritability, anorexia, sweating, sensitivity to light; intolerance of noise |
| More severe symptoms | Depersonalisation; confusion; nausea; delirium; myoclonus (muscular jerking); psychosis. |

Mild withdrawal symptoms may persist for several months; more severe symptoms generally disappear after between 1 and 3 weeks. Benzodiazepine therapy should be withdrawn gradually.

Box 2.3

Symptoms of dependency/ withdrawal associated with long-term benzodiazepine medication

Chlordiazepoxide

Chlordiazepoxide has been used for many years to treat severe disabling anxiety that may or may not be associated with insomnia or psychotic illness. As treatment for anxiety states in adults, the usual dose is 30 mg daily in divided doses. The dose is calculated according to the individual's symptoms and response to the drug: the normal maximum daily dose is 100 g in divided doses. Older and frail clients are usually prescribed half the normal daily dose and for all clients the aim is to give the lowest dose that will control the symptoms. Chlordiazepoxide should not be given when the client is depressed as well as anxious, as in such cases there is a danger of suicide. Short-term use of this agent does not carry a particular risk of dependency, but high-dose therapy over a sustained length of time is more hazardous, especially if the client has a history of addiction or a personality disorder. This product should not be taken in conjunction with other CNS depressant agents and the client should be warned of the possible adverse effects of drowsiness and unsteadiness of gait.

Diazepam

Diazepam is another product that has been in use for a number of years. It is available in a number of formats, including ampoules for injection, rectal preparations and tablets. Diazepam is useful for the short-term treatment of disabling anxiety, or symptoms related to anxiety such as tension headaches. The usual dose for anxiety-related conditions is 2 mg three times daily. It is also an anticonvulsant and reduces muscle spasm and may be used for children to treat night terrors and sleepwalking (see Chapter 4).

A treatment period of no more than 2–3 months is desired to avoid the development of withdrawal symptoms (Box 2.3), physical or psychological dependence. Its use is not advised for clients suffering from depression as there is a increased risk of suicide. It should not be taken in parallel with antihistamines or drugs acting upon the CNS as the effect will be potentiated and undue sedation will result, as will also occur if it is taken with alcohol. In the 1960s and 1970s, this product was treated virtually as a universal panacea and was prescribed very freely by some family doctors. As time passed, patients found that their medication was less benign than had been supposed. Adverse effects of diazepam include, among others, ataxia, confusion, constipation, tremor, urinary retention and alteration of the sex drive.

Lorazepam

This product is used to treat anxiety states and acute mania. It is available in injection or oral formats. As with other benzodiazepines, its use over a sustained period of time is discouraged. If given to an adult as an injection, the dose for acute anxiety is 0.025–0.03 mg per kilogram body weight. It is not recommended for use in children and half of the normal adult dose is used for older clients. Problems associated with sedation, withdrawal and dependency states may occur.

Use of benzodiazepines

Patients need to understand that they may experience drowsiness and incoordination when taking these preparations and they should therefore avoid driving a car or working in hazardous situations. Benzodiazepines are not recommended for pregnant women because there is a risk of fetal malformation if they are taken during the first 12 weeks of pregnancy. If benzodiazepines are taken during advanced pregnancy, the baby may be physiologically dependent, have depressed cardiorespiratory function or be born with impaired hearing.

Benzodiazepines are generally withdrawn gradually to avoid symptoms such as insomnia, depression, nervousness and irritability, sweating and diarrhoea. If the client has been taking high doses of benzodiazepines and the treatment is abruptly halted, confusion, convulsions and psychosis may occur. Overdosage produces an exaggerated form of the pharmacological effect: the client is likely to be drowsy and ataxic. The effects are worse if alcohol has been ingested. There may be cardiovascular or respiratory depression, so pulse, blood pressure and respiratory rate should be monitored. The client may need transfer to acute medical care facilities as intravenous fluids and airway maintenance may be needed to support the cardiovascular and respiratory systems respectively.

Serotonin-1A partial agonists

Serotonin-1A partial agonists such as the buspirone-related compounds – for example, **gepirone, tandospirone, ipsapirone** – may be used for sufferers from GAD. As explained above, these products cause alterations to the sensitivity of neurotransmitter receptors. The development of sustained release formats has meant that patients need to take their medication less often and there is less interaction with alcohol and fewer dependency and withdrawal effects.

Alternative remedies

Kava, which is a relative of the pepper family, has been used in Germany and the USA for the treatment of anxiety and insomnia. Placebo-controlled trials have demonstrated it to be an effective and apparently safe herb for use in short-term anxiety and stress and a range of anxiety disorders such as phobias and generalised anxiety disorder. Kava is thought to work by inhibiting sodium and calcium channels and to interact with the glutamate neurotransmitter system. The use of kava can cause mild gastrointestinal disturbances and skin allergies and it may have an effect upon the benzodiazepine receptor system: Fugh-Berman and Cott (1999) report an instance in which a man who was taking alprazolam, cimetidine and terazosin developed lethargy and disorientation after adding kava to his therapeutic regimen.

Passionflower (*Passiflora incarnata*) is another herb with sedative properties. It is often used in a herbal combination and is believed to be safe. It may work as a partial benzodiazepine agonist. It has been observed to cause an overall reduction in general motor activity in experimental mice but appears to be harmless in man.

Skullcap (*Scutellaria laterifolia*) has been used in combination with passionflower and valerian (see below). In overdose, skullcap causes dizziness, confusion, stupor and convulsive seizures. Some mixed compounds containing skullcap have been reported to cause liver toxicity, although it is not clear which herb was responsible for this effect.

Valerian has long been used as a sedative substance. It has been evaluated along with propranolol and has been found to diminish subjective sensations of anxiety without influencing the physical symptoms associated with it. In contrast, propranolol diminished the physiological effects of arousal. Valerian has been evaluated as relatively safe in overdose. A young person who took a significant overdose of valerian had no changes to the vital signs but suffered fatigue, abdominal cramps, tightness in the chest, lightheadedness and tremor. The patient was treated with activated charcoal and recovered within 24 hours (Fugh-Berman and Cott, 1999). Valerian may produce withdrawal symptoms of tachycardia, tremor and delirium if ceased abruptly.

THE NATURE OF PHOBIA

Phobia is the Greek word for fear, and a range of disorders exist related to specific fears. There are five major subtypes of phobia: agoraphobia, social, animal, situational and blood/injury phobias. Phobic disorders may be mild and appear as little more than an extreme variant of a normal anxiety or may be severe and disabling. Disorders such as social phobia, agoraphobia and other specific phobias will be considered below.

All phobias involve excessive activation of the anxiety response. Interestingly, different types of phobia are thought to evoke different physiological responses: exposure to stimuli such as snakes or heights produces sympathetic stimulation – the characteristic fright, fight or flight response – whereas blood/injury phobia seems to evoke excessive parasympathetic activity, resulting in fainting due to the hypotension and bradycardia of vagal stimulation (Kendler *et al.*, 2001). These same researchers undertook a study of phobias in twin males that has led to the suggestion that agoraphobia and social phobia are probably more influenced by family environment than are other forms of phobia.

Specific phobias involve an unreasonable fear response to a given situation, be it flying in an aeroplane; procedures involving needles, injections or blood; fear of spiders or animals or, in the case of some women, tocophobia – fear of childbirth

Tocophobia

This phobia affects a small number of women, who have an illogical dread of giving birth, being convinced that they will die in the process. The dread of childbirth generally involves excessive fear of the pain of delivery, and may begin in adolescence. The affected woman may have a normal sexual relationship but is likely to take excessive care with contraception, possibly using several methods simultaneously. Some women who do become pregnant seek delivery by caesarean section in order to avoid the need to give birth vaginally. If they are obliged to give birth vaginally, there may be impaired bonding with the baby or, occasionally, the woman may subsequently suffer depression or PTSD (see below). In some cases, tocophobia has been found to follow rape or childhood sexual abuse, or it may be associated with a previous traumatic delivery. The condition may lead some women to seek surgical sterilisation to avoid all risk of pregnancy. Hofberg and Brockington (2000) describe an interesting series of cases of women with this condition.

Social phobia

This is thought to be the third most common mental health disorder after depression and alcoholism (Van Ameringen et al., 2001). People with social phobia complain of feelings of embarrassment and a fear of coping with social situations or other people's performance expectations. When someone with social phobia is put into what is for them a threatening situation, they experience a profound 'fright or flight' response: dry mouth, palpitations, tremors, sweating, abdominal cramps, diarrhoea, inability to think clearly and uncontrollable blushing. Social phobia may cause a change in habit in order to avoid the social stressors; for example, the sufferer may avoid eating, writing or speaking in public in case they are the subject of critical comment. There may be a profound fear of rejection, general inability to behave assertively, lack of social skills and self esteem and an overall detrimental effect upon the lifestyle.

Mendlowicz and Stein (2000) suggest that social phobia was underrecognised until the 1980s, being mistaken for ordinary social shyness, but that in fact the condition produces significant detrimental effects upon the sufferer's quality of life. Subthreshold social phobia is a less disabling form of social phobia in which the individual assiduously avoids a specific challenge such as public speaking or meeting strangers. Social phobia is thought particularly to affect men who have attained a degree of intellectual social and occupational success. It is thought that mothers with social phobia and anxiety disorders tend to have children who are particularly shy or who later go on to develop social phobia themselves (Cooper and Eke, 1999; Lieb et al., 2000). The development of social phobia during adolescence or young adulthood is associated with the later development of depressive disorders (Stein et al., 2001). A client with social phobia may also suffer from panic disorder, major depressive episodes, alcohol or substance abuse.

Despite this, researchers suggest that social phobia is often missed when a client seeks medical advice (Pande et al., 1999). These authors suggest that people with social phobia frequently seek medical help but are not always appropriately treated. Subthreshold social phobia has been described as predominantly affecting unmarried females who have fewer educational attainments and a lower occupational income.

Serotonin lack appears to be involved with the development of social phobia. It has also been suggested that sufferers have a low dopamine-2-receptor binding ability (Schneier *et al.*, 2000). Specific serotonin reuptake inhibitors (SSRIs) such as **paroxetine** have been used successfully in the treatment of social phobia (Baldwin *et al.*, 1999). Sufferers have also been reported to benefit from treatment with the SSRI **fluvoxamine**. Benzodiazepine anxiolytics and MAOIs have also been used to treat clients with the condition. Cognitive-behavioural therapy in combination with pharmacotherapy has been found to be helpful.

Key point ▶

> Social phobia has detrimental effects upon the sufferer's lifestyle and is associated with the development of depressive conditions. It appears that there is a familial link.

Fluvoxamine has been found to be helpful in the treatment of social phobia, although it is more commonly ordered for clients suffering from depressive illness or OCD (see below). The normal dose is between 100–200 mg daily, with the lowest dose being used that achieves relief from the symptoms. The drug can cause insomnia, generalised weakness and sexual dysfunction in men. If clients suddenly cease taking fluvoxamine, withdrawal symptoms such as headache, nausea, paraesthesia ('pins and needles'), anxiety and dizziness may occur. Overdosage is treated with activated charcoal.

Moclobemide, in a maximum dose of 600 mg daily in two divided doses, is also recommended for clients suffering from social phobia. Treatment is usually commenced at 300 mg daily and then increased to achieve therapeutic levels. The treatment may be of long duration, as social phobia is a persistent condition. Moclobemide is a reversible monoamine oxidase inhibitor (MOAI), so interaction with SSRIs and tricyclic antidepressants may occur. The reversible nature of this drug usually means that dietary restriction of tyramine-containing foods is not needed unless the client is particularly sensitive to tyramine (see Chapter 3, in which tricyclic antidepressants are discussed). Moclobemide can produce a range of undesirable effects, such as sleep disturbances, agitation, anxiety, dizziness, restlessness, irritability, headache, dry mouth and gastrointestinal symptoms such as diarrhoea or constipation. Overdosage may produce agitation, aggressiveness and other behavioural changes. If no other substances have been taken, the effects of moclobemide overdose are usually not life-threatening.

Paroxetine may be given for panic disorder, social anxiety disorder or social phobia. To control the symptoms of panic disorder, the client may be commenced on 10 mg daily and the dose adjusted upwards to the recommended dose of 40 mg daily For social anxiety disorder or social phobia, a dose of 20 mg daily is commenced and may be gradually adjusted upwards to a maximum of 50 mg daily. Stein *et al.*

(1998) undertook a randomised controlled trial. The results suggested that 11 weeks of treatment with paroxetine produced significant improvements in symptoms and disability from social phobia.

Paroxetine is not licensed for use in children. When used for older clients, plasma levels may need to be monitored to avoid the accumulation of toxic levels. Adverse effects of paroxetine include sleepiness, nausea, dryness of the mouth, sweating, tremor, weakness, sexual dysfunction, dizziness, alteration of bowel function and decreased appetite. Paroxetine is thought to be relatively safe in overdose; common effects include nausea, vomiting, tremor, drowsiness, dry mouth, dilated pupils, irritability and sweating. Use of activated charcoal helps to delay absorption of ingested paroxetine.

Phenelzine may be used for clients with anxiety mixed with depression or phobic symptoms. Heimberg *et al.* (1998) recommend the use of phenelzine with cognitive behavioural therapy as treatment for social phobia. The preparation is usually given orally in a dose of 15 mg three times daily. For the majority, this dosage results in an improvement within a week, otherwise the dose may be increased to a maximum of 15 mg three times daily to achieve control of the symptoms, and then reduced to achieve a maintenance dose.

Phenelzine is not licensed for children under 16 years of age. It may be prescribed for older clients, although postural hypotension may make its use problematic and it is not appropriate for clients who are already receiving medication for cerebrovascular conditions or congestive heart failure. Because phenelzine interacts with many drugs and older clients are more likely to be prescribed a range of medicines (polypharmacy), a special watch for drug interactions is needed. Common adverse effects include dizziness, drowsiness, weakness and fatigue, oedema, nausea, vomiting, drying of the mouth, constipation, insomnia, blurring of the vision and postural hypotension. Overdosage of phenelzine may be lethal. Hypomania and euphoria may precede coma. The blood pressure may either rise, causing a risk of stroke, or hypotension may occur, causing cardiovascular collapse.

Sertraline is also used for clients with mixed anxiety and depression. It is usually given in a daily dose of 5 mg in a single daily dose. There may be signs of an improvement in the client's condition after 7 days, although usually it takes 2–4 weeks for the full effect of treatment to be seen. It appears acceptable for treatment for older clients but its safe use is not proven in children. Common adverse effects include nausea, diarrhoea, anorexia, dyspepsia, tremor, dizziness, sleep disturbances, sweating, dry mouth and sexual dysfunction. Sertraline is thought to be fairly safe in overdose if taken alone.

In the USA, Pande *et al.* (1999) have investigated the use of **gabapentin,** which is more commonly used as a non-benzodiazepine anticonvulsant. The mode of action of gabapentin is not at present well understood. It is not thought to work on the benzodiazepine receptor system nor to have a direct influence upon the action of serotonin in the CNS. It was found that, for sufferers from social phobia, gabapentin produced anxiolytic effects comparable to those attained by the use of benzodiazepines, without the adverse effects associated with that group of drugs. Their findings have led Pande *et al.* to suggest that social phobia is likely to be caused by multiple mechanisms, rather than primarily via the benzodiazepine receptor or serotonin neurotransmitter systems and to propose gabapentin as an effective medication that may be found to be acceptable as treatment for sufferers from social phobia. Adverse effects appear to be mild but include dizziness, dryness of the mouth and, on occasions, sleepiness, nausea, flatulence and reduced libido.

Panic disorder

Sufferers from panic disorder experience unexpected recurrent feelings of intense panic with no identifiable logical cause followed by a period of deep concern about the attack or fear of experience of a recurrence. The sufferer may endure a run of attacks on a daily basis for a week and then have little or no recurrence for months. Symptoms associated with panic disorder reflect an extreme picture of the arousal response: rapid pulse or palpitations; trembling; sweating; feelings of difficulty in breathing; a sense of choking; pain in the chest; nausea or abdominal discomfort; numbness or tingling, often of the lips hands and feet; feelings of unreality or lightheadedness; feelings of losing sanity or control or a sense of impending death. Panic attacks commonly accompany agoraphobia, the fear of being alone in crowds, public transport or open spaces.

Panic disorder seems to be a lifetime problem that requires treatment. It may be associated with hyperventilation syndrome (see Chapter 8). Pharmacological treatment of panic disorder is thought to work via the serotonin system by desensitising pathways between the amygdala, the hypothalamus and the brain stem.

Key point ▶

> The symptoms of panic disorder are the result of excessive activation of the sympathetic nervous system and chemical imbalance due to an inappropriate ventilatory response.

The patient with panic attacks may be treated with imipramine 2.25 mg/ kg body weight per day for 6 months. Sufferers may also respond to treatment with clonazepam, sertraline, paroxetine, fluoxetine or clomipramine (Mendlowicz and Stein, 2000). The benzodiazepines **alprazolam clonazepam** or **diazepam** may also be given. Psychosocial therapies are thought to be helpful because they operate at the level of the prefrontal cortex and hippocampus to reduce the cognitive elements of fear (Gorman *et al.*, 2000).

Post-traumatic stress disorder

Post-traumatic stress disorder has been described in soldiers after military campaigns as well in as survivors and witnesses of disasters and violent crime. Subsequently, sufferers may feel helpless or excessively fearful, or have a sense of horror. They may experience recurrent flash-backs or intrusive feelings related to the original shocking event and a sense of depersonalisation and loss of involvement in activities that were previously enjoyed. In addition, there is a collection of sensations consistent with abnormal arousal: there may be a partial loss of recall of the trigger event, sleep disorders, emotional lability, exaggerated alarm response, or difficulty in thinking, concentrating or maintaining usual relationships.

The physical effects of PTSD include increased heart and respiratory rate and elevated blood pressure and increased urinary levels of the stress hormones noradrenaline (norepinephrine) and cortisol. Additionally, there is increased skin conductance (an indicator of stress), increased muscle tone and a chronic increase in plasma thyroxine levels, consistent with the effects of chronic stress. Sufferers from PTSD have altered sleep patterns, with loss of total sleep time, increased time taken to fall asleep, delayed rapid-eye-movement sleep, increased waking during sleep and vivid nightmares occurring earlier than usual during the sleep cycle (Walker, 1996).

- Altered lateralisation of brain functioning possibly causing intrusive ideation; increased anxious watchfulness and emotional blunting
- Biochemical alteration of the cells of the hippocampus, possibly due to chronic overproduction of cortisol and resulting in altered memory processing
- Alteration of the normal relationships between the sympathetic nervous system and the adrenal medulla and the pituitary gland and the adrenal cortex respectively, possibly resulting in paranoid behaviour
- Alteration of noradrenaline production in the CNS, resulting in overstimulation of the locus ceruleus and exacerbation of the symptoms of post-traumatic stress disorder.

Box 2.4

Possible biological causes of the symptoms of post-traumatic stress disorder (Walker, 1996)

Specific serotonin reuptake inhibitors such as fluoxetine, sertraline, paroxetine or fluvoxamine have been found to be helpful in improving the symptoms.

Experimental work with cholecystokinin (CCK)-4, which is known to interact with CCK-B receptors in the brain stem, has been undertaken. The CCK-4 was observed to be associated with a flashback experience for an American patient suffering from PTSD who had been shot in the stomach 4 years previously. This has led to the suggestion that brain-stem CCK-B receptors may be involved in the pathophysiology of flashbacks associated with PTSD (Kellner *et al.*, 1998).

Post-traumatic stress disorder seems to occur when there are altera-tions in the balance of activity between neural and endocrine struc-tures governing the normal anxiety response.

◄ **Key point**

Obsessive–compulsive disorder

Obsessive–compulsive disorder is a syndrome in which the quality of the sufferer's life is adversely influenced by intrusive and inappropriate thoughts and actions that are respectively termed obsessions and compulsions. **Obsessions** are thoughts, images or impulses preceding an action. They are commonly related to the fear of causing harm to another through failure to complete some important set of actions. Obsessive thoughts may centre on notions of infection or contamination, a need for precision in an activity or arrangement of objects, religious ideation or concerns about bodily functioning. Such thoughts are often accompanied by feelings of shame and fear. Sufferers know that the ideas come from within themselves, rather than from some outside agency, as is the case in schizophrenia.

Compulsions are observable actions, usually undertaken in response to the original obsessive thoughts. Compulsions may include cleaning or washing rituals, counting, checking or arranging, or collecting things. The compulsive action is commonly undertaken so as to ward off some potential disaster that would otherwise occur as a result of the sufferer's lack of attention. Usually this process involves the creation of rigid rules so as to avoid the dreaded occurrence. Because the rituals are not logical, the sufferer usually realises at some level that the strategies are inappropriate, and this tends to cause distress and anxiety and a redoubled effort with the rituals. The illness is thus likely to spiral out of control so that it comes to dominate the person's life.

Key point ▶

> The sufferer from OCD is generally aware that there is no logical basis for his/her feelings and actions but cannot control them, nor the anxiety generated as a result.

Obsessive–compulsive disorder often develops in childhood or young adulthood. Most of us probably engage upon some ritualistic set of activities that is irrationally aimed at preventing an adverse event. Children often avoid cracks in pavements, we may return several times to check the front door or that the car is locked because of sudden doubts that security has been compromised. OCD has been found to be quite common in the population, occurring in 1 in 50 adults and 1 in 200 children (Stahl, 1996), and may be encountered in any social class, racial group or culture. In some, there is a clear trigger event that precipitated the condition; other people slowly develop OCD for no apparent reason.

The biology of obsessive–compulsive disorder

Positron-emission tomography (PET) scanning of the brains of clients with OCD has demonstrated abnormal neuronal activity within the basal ganglia and possible abnormal communication with the orbito-frontal cortex. There is evidence that OCD runs in families and has

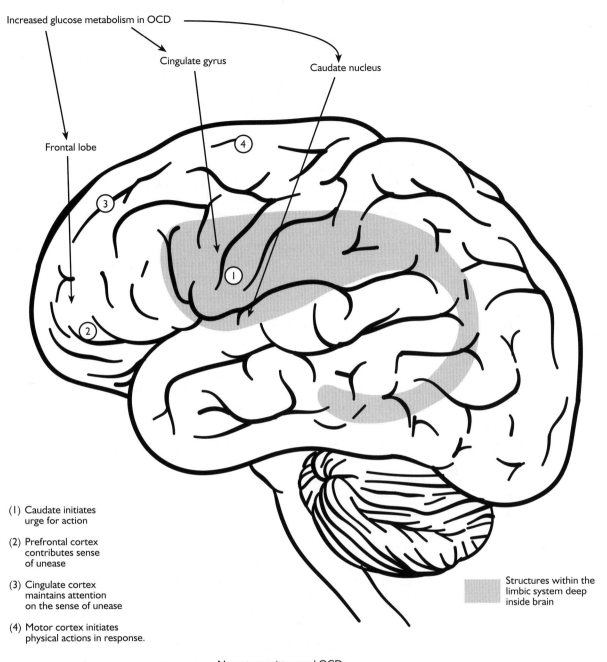

Increased glucose metabolism in OCD

Cingulate gyrus

Caudate nucleus

Frontal lobe

(1) Caudate initiates
urge for action

(2) Prefrontal cortex
contributes sense
of unease

(3) Cingulate cortex
maintains attention
on the sense of unease

(4) Motor cortex initiates
physical actions in response.

Structures within the
limbic system deep
inside brain

Neurotransmitters and OCD:

Serotonin mediates washing and danger avoidance behaviours

OCD — altered cerebral serotonin metabolism

Figure 2.8

Mechanisms involved in obsessive–compulsive disorder

some genetic basis. It has been suggested that OCD occurs because of altered neuronal or neurotransmitter activity and that some disorder of the basal ganglia is responsible. It is likely that the condition is caused in part at least by a disorder of the serotonin neurotransmitter system. Observation of the improvement of the symptoms of OCD in clients receiving treatment with SSRIs has promoted the understanding that obsessional behaviour is linked with serotonin deficits at the synapses (Figure 2.8).

A proportion of OCD sufferers are unaffected by SSRI therapy or have OCD with no observable defect in the serotonin system. Experimental use of substances, such as amfetamine, L-dopa and bromocriptine, which influence dopamine pathways in the brain, have been found to produce obsessive–compulsive behaviours similar to those that occur in OCD. Cocaine also produces similar effects. Conditions such as Tourette's syndrome, in which the person suffers compulsive motor movements ('tics') and compulsive vocalisation, often of obscenities, are known to be associated with an abnormality of dopamine within the basal ganglia, and Tourette's sufferers are known to have obsessions and compulsions. Neuroleptic drugs that block dopamine-A receptors, if given in conjunction with SSRI medication (see below), can provide effective treatment for OCD or for Tourette's syndrome in clients who do not respond to SSRIs alone. There is therefore a theory that OCD, particularly that linked with Tourette's syndrome, is an entity associated with imbalances in both the serotonin and dopamine mechanisms. This would result in an excess of dopamine, which is associated with the characteristic manifestations of OCD and Tourette's syndrome.

Key point ▶

> Obsessive–compulsive disorder appears to be caused by alterations in the balance of serotonin and/or dopamine.

Pharmacological treatment

A number of clients who have OCD also have depression, so over the years the effect of antidepressant treatment upon obsessive–compulsive symptoms have been noted. The use of the tricyclic antidepressant clomipramine was noted in the 1980s to be beneficial. At first, this was thought to be due to the antidepressant effect but eventually it became clear that clomipramine, a potent serotonin-reuptake inhibiting agent (SSRI), had a specific effect upon obsessive–compulsive symptoms. In order for an antidepressant to be effective against the symptoms of OCD, the agent must either influence dopamine, by diminishing the concentration at the synapses, or increase serotonin concentrations. Antidepressants that block noradrenaline uptake have no effect upon obsessive–compulsive symptoms.

The dose of SSRI to treat OCD is significantly greater than that used to treat depression. In addition, the length of time needed to achieve therapeutic concentrations is much longer – 12 weeks or more compared with the 4–8 weeks needed to obtain an antidepressant effect.

Despite the treatability of OCD with clomipramine and SSRIs, the disorder tends to recur once the medication is discontinued. It is thought that different mechanisms occur when OCD is treated by SSRIs in comparison with the use of the same agent to treat depression.

> Obsessive–compulsive disorder can be successfully treated with SSRIs given at a higher dose than that used for depression. The treatment effect takes longer to achieve and symptoms may return on cessation of medication.

◀ *Key point*

Not all OCD sufferers respond to SSRI treatment, which has led pharmaceutical chemists to develop other strategies for increasing the concentration of serotonin at the synapses. SSRIs work by blocking the reuptake of serotonin, which is released from the presynaptic vesicles. If there was insufficient serotonin released into the synapse in the first place, there would be no serotonin to retain, so inhibition of reuptake by the use of SSRIs would not work. This reasoning has led to the development of combination therapy.

Combination therapy to enhance serotonin levels in the synapses

If serotonin depletion is part of the problem, there is a need to build up stores so that sufficient concentration within the synapses can be regained. If the activity of serotonin-secreting neurones can be reduced, then the neurotransmitter stores are less rapidly used up and can gradually be augmented as naturally occurring tryptophan is used to make more serotonin. This is achieved by the use of a serotonin (5-$HT1_A$) partial agonist such as buspirone to slow the responsiveness of the neurone (and 'save' serotonin), combined with the use of a SSRI to extend the dwell time of serotonin in the synapses. If the serotonin problem is due to a failure of the presynaptic neurone to release the transmitter, this can be remedied by the use of an agent, such as fenfluramine, that 'drives' the presynaptic neurone to release serotonin, which can then be retained in the synapses by the use of SSRIs.

If the problem is due to a failure of the mechanism of the postsynaptic receptor, such that each molecule of serotonin is so avidly taken up by the postsynaptic receptor that an insufficient concentration of serotonin is left in the synapses, a drug that suppresses (downregulates) the postsynaptic receptors may be helpful. The aim of this is to reduce the number of postsynaptic receptors but for those remaining to be resensitised so that fewer molecules of serotonin can be used to greater effect to stimulate the postsynaptic neurone. The result is once more that serotonin levels in the synapse are optimised and the symptoms, whether of depression, OCD or panic disorder, are reduced. Examples of such serotonin-2 antagonist/reuptake inhibitors (SARIs) are trazodone and nefazodone.

Combination therapy is thought to work by:

- reducing serotonin usage via the use of serotonin partial agonists
- driving the presynaptic neurone to release more serotonin
- increasing the sensitivity and reducing the number of postsynaptic receptors (downregulation).

As indicated earlier, the symptoms of OCD due to synaptic serotonin depletion can be also be treated by the use of neuroleptic agents, which block dopamine receptors and thus alter the dopamine/serotonin balance within the synapses. This is sometimes beneficial for clients whose symptoms have schizoid characteristics. Benzodiazepine agents such as clonazepam may be helpful in that they enhance the effect of SSRIs in addition to reducing the anxiety-related symptoms that are a feature of OCD. Agents with potential for development in the treatment of OCD include nefazodone, which is a weak SSRI and also influences serotonin-2 receptors, venlafaxine, which influences serotonin and noradrenaline reuptake, and risperidone, which inhibits serotonin-2 and dopamine-2 receptors.

Pharmacological treatment is of course only part of the treatment for OCD: clients need psychological support and the use of positive examples to enable them to develop functional ways of interacting. Behavioural and or group therapy and other cognitive interventions beyond the scope of this book form equally important strategies for helping the client learn to cope with this disabling condition. A useful overview of OCD and useful treatment modalities may be found in Gournay, 1998.

Figure 2.9

Drug modalities for the treatment of obsessive–compulsive disorder

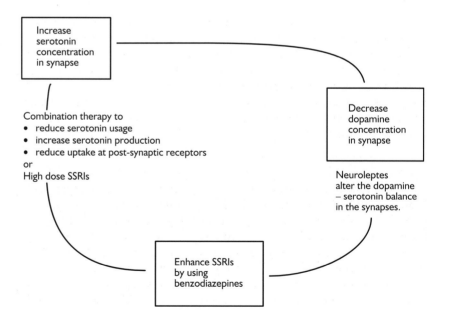

Increase serotonin concentration in synapse

Combination therapy to
- reduce serotonin usage
- increase serotonin production
- reduce uptake at post-synaptic receptors
or
High dose SSRIs

Decrease dopamine concentration in synapse

Neuroleptes alter the dopamine – serotonin balance in the synapses.

Enhance SSRIs by using benzodiazepines

CASE STUDY 2.3   MAGGIE, A PATIENT WITH OBSESSIVE–COMPULSIVE DISORDER

Read this case study and then attempt to answer the questions that follow.

Maggie Obatu is a 36-year-old woman. She has two children aged 8 and 10 years and has lived for a number of years happily with her husband in the same house. Her family doctor has referred her for an assessment after her husband took her to the surgery.

Maggie has had the same job in an accounts office for the last 5 years but over the last 18 months she has been seen by the manager on several occasions because of her poor timekeeping in the mornings. This is the history she gives.

She has gradually become increasingly concerned about her ability to keep the house clean, feeling that, if she fails in this responsibility, her children may get meningitis and be dead within hours. During the late evening she therefore cleans and scours the house, particularly the bathroom, so that, when the children get ready for school, they don't pick up germs from the wash basin. Her cleaning activities revolve particularly around intensive efforts to clean the plughole and the overflow, which she may repeat eight to 10 times each evening. Her lateness in the mornings stems from a ritual she undertakes that involves touching each corner of the front door four times, once for each member of the family. She then has to repeat the ritual four times in the belief that, should she fail to do this sufficient times, a member of her family will die. The activity has to be completed perfectly, without faltering. As she is worried that she might forget where she has got to, she often has to start all over from scratch, which makes her late for work and increasingly anxious. Her husband Leroy is concerned for her welfare, and also because their children make fun of her, which makes the whole situation worse.

1. Is there likely to be a predisposing cause for Maggie's condition?
2. What help will Maggie need to overcome this condition?
3. Maggie is in the first instance prescribed SSRIs and group therapy. What should she know about her treatment?

SUMMARY

Anxiety is a normal arousal mechanism allowing an effective response to challenge. In health, the stimulator and suppresser neurotransmitters remain in balance. The arousal response involves neuroendocrine mechanisms: these become unbalanced in the anxiety-related disorders, which may significantly detract from a person's quality of life. The choice of treatment for anxiety-related disorders is determined, among other considerations, by the chronicity of the condition and whether depression is also present.

There is some interesting evidence to suggest that OCD responds to some hallucinogenic substances. Compounds such as lysergic acid diethylamide (LSD); psilocybin (the chemical in *Psilocybe*, 'magic mushrooms') and mescaline (the hallucinogenic substance in peyote cacti) are all agonists of serotonin-2A receptors. Perrine (1999) reports the case of a 34-year-old man who had suffered from OCD since he was 6 years old. This client reported an improvement of his OCD symptoms, including ritualistic washing activities and compulsive counting, after he experimented with mescaline and

Box 2.5

'Zoned out' and free of obsessive–compulsive disorder?

psilocybin respectively. He had now begun a 4-year course of daily psilocybin mushrooms and his OCD symptoms had improved! Because psilocybin causes the serotonin-2A receptor system to downregulate and therefore to become less responsive to serotonin in the synapses, tolerance occurs, so the patient benefits from the reduction of his OCD but is denied the hallucinogenic effects of the magic mushrooms!

REFERENCES AND FURTHER READING

Baldwin, D., Bobes, J., Stein, D.J. *et al.* (1999) Paroxetine in social phobia/social anxiety disorder. Randomised, double-blind, placebo-controlled study. Paroxetine Study Group. *British Journal of Psychiatry*, **175**, 120–126.

Carlson, N.R. (2001) *Physiology of behaviour*, 7th edn. Allyn & Bacon, Boston, MA.

Cates, M., Wells, B.G. and Thatcher, W. (1996) Anxiety disorders. In: *Textbook of Therapeutics: Drug and Disease Management*, eds E.T. Herfindal and D.R. Gourley. Williams & Wilkins, Baltimore, MD, ch. 53.

Cooper, P.J. and Eke, M. (1999) Childhood shyness and maternal social phobia: a community study. *British Journal of Psychiatry* 174, 439–443.

Fugh-Berman, A. and Cott, J.M. (1999) Dietary supplements and natural products as psychotherapeutic agents. *Psychosomatic Medicine*, **61**, 712.

Garcia, C., Micallef, J., Dubreuil, D. *et al.* (2000) Effects of lorazepam on emotional reactivity, performance and vigilance in subjects with high or low anxiety. *Journal of Clinical Psychopharmacology*, **20**, 226–233.

Gorman, J.M., Kent, J.M., Sullivan, G.M. and Coplan, J.D. (2000) Neuroanatomical hypothesis of panic disorder, revised. *American Journal of Psychiatry*, **157**, 493–505.

Gournay, K. (1998) Obsessive compulsive disorder: nature and treatment. *Nursing Standard*, **13**, 46–54.

Heimberg, R.G., Liebowitz, M.R., Hope, D.A. *et al.* (1998) Cognitive behavioural group therapy vs. phenelzine therapy for social phobia: 12 week outcome. *Archives of General Psychiatry*, **55**, 1133–1141.

Hofberg, K. and Brockington, I (2000) Tokophobia: an unreasoning dread of childbirth: a series of 26 cases. *British Journal of Psychiatry*, **176**, 83–85

Jacobs-Rebhun, S., Schnurr, P.P., Friedman, M.J. *et al.* (2000) Posttraumatic stress disorder and sleep difficulty. *American Journal of Psychiatry*, **157**, 1525–1526.

Kellner, M., Levengood, R., Yehuda, R. and Wiedemann, K. (1998) Provocation of a post traumatic flashback by cholecystokinin tetrapeptide? *American Journal of Psychiatry*, **155**, 1299.

Kendler, K.S., Myers, J.M.S., Prescott, C.A. and Neale, M.C. (2001) The genetic epidemiology of irrational fears and phobias in men. *Archives of General Psychiatry*, **58**, 256–257.

Lieb, R., Wittchen, H.-U., Hofler, M. *et al.* (2000) Parental psychopathology, parenting styles and the risk of social phobia in offspring: a prospective-longitudinal community study. *Archives of General Psychiatry*, **57**, 859–866.

Mendlowicz, M.V. and Stein, M.B. (2000) Quality of life in individuals with anxiety disorders. *American Journal of Psychiatry*, **157**, 669–682.

Pande, A.C., Davidson, J.R.T., Jefferson, J.W. *et al.* (1999) Treatment of social phobia with gabapentin: a placebo-controlled study. *Journal of Clinical Psychopharmacology*, **19**, 341–348.

Perrine, D.M. (1999) Hallucinogens and obsessive–compulsive disorder. *American Journal of Psychiatry*, **156**, 1123.

Rickels, K., Pollack, M.H., Sheehan, D.V. and Haskins, J.T. (2000) Efficacy of extended-release venlafaxine in nondepressed outpatients with generalised anxiety disorder. *American Journal of Psychiatry*, **157**, 968–974.

Rijnders, R., Laman, D.M. and van Diujn, H. (2000) Cyproheptadine for posttraumatic nightmares. *American Journal of Psychiatry*, **157**, 1523–1525.

Schneier, E.R., Liebowitz, M., Abi-Dargham, A. *et al.* (2000) Low dopamine D$_2$ receptor binding potential in social phobia. *American Journal of Psychiatry*, **157**, 457–459.

Selye H, (1976) *The Stress of Life*. McGraw-Hill, New York.

Stahl, S.M (1996) *Essential Psychopharmacology: Neuroscientific Basis and Practical Applications*. Cambridge University Press, Cambridge.

Stein, M.B., Fuetsch, M.M., Muller, N. *et al.* (2001) Social anxiety disorder and the risk of depression: a prospective community study of adolescents and young adults. *Archives of General Psychiatry*, **58**, 251–256.

Stein, M.B., Liebowitz, M.R., Lydiard, R.B. *et al.* (1998) Paroxetine treatment of generalised social phobia (social anxiety disorder): a randomised controlled trial. *Journal of the American Medical Association*, **280**, 708–713.

Van Ameringen, M.A., Lane, R.M., Walker, J.R. *et al.* (2001) Sertraline treatment of generalised social phobia: a 20 week double-blind placebo-controlled study. *American Journal of Psychiatry*, **158**, 275–291.

Walker, A. (1996) *Biological Changes in PTSD*. http://york39.ncl.ac.uk/www/PTSDAlison.html

Yerkes, R.M. and Dodson, J.D. (1908) The relationship of strength of stimulus to rapidity of habit formations. *Journal of Comparative Neurology and Psychology*, **18**, 459–458.

Websites

Obsessive–compulsive disorder: http://www.1-obsessive–compulsive-disorder.com/

Phobias: http://www.phobialist.com; http://www.phobiascured.com

SELF-TEST QUESTIONS

Identify the correct statements in the following questions. For each question, some, all or no options may be correct.

1. Which of the following are involved with the chronic stress response:
   a. gamma-aminobutyric acid (GABA)
   b. corticotrophic releasing factor
   c. acetylcholine
   d. noradrenaline (norepinephrine)

2. A naturally occurring calming substance produced within the central nervous system is:
   a. serotonin
   b. benzodiazepine
   c. gamma-aminobutyric acid (GABA)
   d. corticotropin (corticotrophin)

3. Benzodiazepine anxiolytics have which of the following properties:
   a. produce muscle relaxation

   b.   have an anticonvulsant effect

   c.   produce a rapid sense of wellbeing

   d.   promote sleep

4.   Partial serotonin agonists treat anxiety by which of the following mechanisms:

   a.   they act like serotonin to stimulate mood

   b.   they prevent downregulation of serotonin receptors

   c.   the rebalancing of serotonin at the synapses produces a slow anxiolytic effect

   d.   readjustment of serotonin at the synapses rapidly reduces anxiety

5.   A client with general anxiety disorder may be treated with which of the following:

   a.   long-term benzodiazepine anxiolytics

   b.   short-term tricyclic antidepressants

   c.   short-term benzodiazepine anxiolytics

   d.   partial serotonin agonists

6.   Which of the following are common symptoms of post-traumatic stress disorder?

   a.   sleep disturbance

   b.   increased muscle tone

   c.   intrusive flashbacks

   d.   diminished concentration

7.   Which of the following statements are true about phobic disorders?

   a.   agoraphobia and social phobia may be influenced by some factors within family life

   b.   women with tocophobia can be helped if they experience a natural birth

   c.   fear of spiders (arachnophobia) evokes excessive reaction within the sympathetic nervous system

   d.   clients with fear of blood and needles may faint as a result of slow pulse and low blood pressure

8.   Which of the following are features of obsessive–compulsive disorder?

   a.   sufferers think that their ideas originate from some source outside themselves

   b.   obsessive thoughts often revolve around the notion of harm to others resulting from a failure to observe precautions

   c.   compulsions are actions carried out in response to obsessive thoughts

   d.   it primarily affects people from well-educated, affluent groups

9.   Which of the following treatments may help a client with obsessive–compulsive disorder?

   a.   dopamine enhancers such as bromocriptine and behavioural therapy

   b.   clomipramine and group therapy

   c.   serotonin partial agonists such as buspirone and SSRIs

   d.   paroxetine and a SARI such as trazodone

10. A client suffers from panic attacks. Which of the following statements are correct?
    a. the symptoms are those of an inappropriate arousal response
    b. it rarely poses a risk to physical health
    c. chest pain, nausea or abdominal discomfort may be present
    d. the condition is self-limiting

3

ALTERED MOOD: DEPRESSION AND BIPOLAR DISORDERS

INTRODUCTION

The interaction between mind, body and the environment contributes to the mood, or affect. The nervous and the endocrine systems form the communication systems linking somatic tissues with the brain, where the information is interpreted and mood is influenced. It is therefore not surprising that many people with disordered affect initially seek medical help for what they perceive to be a physical problem. Shaw *et al.* (1999), investigating how Afro-Caribbeans and white Europeans sought help for anxiety and depressive illness, found that the majority of the people in their sample had presented with psychosomatic symptoms. However, in contrast, there was a view that the 'tablets' offered by their family doctors were not what they needed; that they did not have an illness and that the doctor would not be interested in their problem. The same authors found that the prevalence of anxiety and depression in both ethnic groups was comparable and that a significant proportion of the subjects of the study used self-treatment with herbal remedies. In this chapter, the pathophysiology of depression and its treatment with pharmacological and herbal or dietary products will be considered. Following this, bipolar conditions, when the mood fluctuates from dejection to elation, will be discussed.

DEPRESSION

Disorders of affect may be described as **unipolar**, in which the mood is characterised by feelings of sadness and inadequacy, or **bipolar**, when the sadness alternates with hyperactivity and a general 'high' feeling. Unipolar depressive illness will be considered first.

Depression is a commonly occurring condition that blights a consid-erable proportion of some people's lives. Sir Winston Churchill is reported to have likened his recurrent depressed moods to being followed by a 'black dog'; others have likened the experience to living at constant risk of slipping into a metaphorical steep pit with slippery sides and indescribable misery at the bottom. Health professionals are not exempt from depression: the reader is directed to the work of Rippere and Williams (1985) for powerful insights into experiences reported by mental health workers.

It is part of the normal human state to feel sometimes happy, sometimes sad. This range of moods can usually be attributed to specific triggers, although we may find ourselves feeling good or bad without a specific cause. The state of depression is marked by a consistent lowering of the mood, with an inability to feel pleasure (anhedonia) and general feelings of hopelessness. There may simply be a feeling of loss of interest in everyday activities. Depression may occur from childhood onwards, although it is probably under-reported in childhood and old age. In childhood, adolescence and old age depressed behaviour may be wrongly interpreted as normal for that age group: young people may be misinterpreted as sulking and with older people there may be a view that sadness is an unavoidable part of life because of the losses that occur in the later parts of the lifespan. In general, disorders of affect are the result of an interaction between the individual's environment and his/her genetic makeup and predisposition to suffer disruption of mood through activation of the stress response within the nervous and endocrine systems. There appears to be a relationship between the frequency of stressful life events and the incidence of affective disorders. (See Chapter 2 for a discussion of the stress response.)

> At certain points in the lifespan, the symptoms of depressive illness may be confused with 'normal' behaviour and remain undiagnosed.

◄ *Key point*

A range of symptoms is associated with depression and an episode is defined as a major depression when five or more of the symptoms listed in Table 3.1 are present most of the day, most days, for at least 2 weeks.

Sleep and appetite may be increased or diminished and the normal sleep architecture is lost, with the sufferer commonly waking at intervals during the night or waking early and then being unable to go back to sleep. It appears that the sleep architecture itself is disrupted, with premature episodes of rapid-eye-movement (REM) sleep and abnormal slow-wave sleep. The patient may appear agitated, displaying restless activity such as pacing or other repetitive mannerisms, or, if psychomotor retardation is present, there may be slowness or absence of speech or reduced body movement. The condition may develop over days or weeks and persist for 6 months or more if not treated. Some people suffer from recurrent major depression throughout their lives. Following the initial episode, 50–80% of patients will experience further depression at some stage (Judd *et al.*, 1991). The findings from

---

- Consistently feeling 'low' (either self-reported or apathy noted by others)
- Loss of interest or pleasure in usual activities
- Consistent alteration of appetite or increase or reduction (more than 5% change) in body weight over a month
- Altered sleep, either reduced or increased
- Altered psychomotor activity, either agitation or reduced activity (retardation)
- Feeling of fatigue or reduced energy
- Feelings of inappropriate guilt or unworthiness
- Impaired cognition: reports of difficulty with thinking or concentrating or undue indecisiveness
- Preoccupation with death; thoughts of suicide

If five or more of these features are present with no organic cause or clear predisposing event, and if hallucinations, delusions or schizophrenia are absent, this constitutes a major depressive episode.

Table 3.1

Changes from normal functioning associated with depressive illness.

the NORDEP-1 trial suggest that women benefit more than men from antidepressant therapy (Malt *et al.*, 1999).

Key point ▶ | For some people, depressive illness may be a recurrent problem throughout their lives.

Dysthymia

While practising in the community, the mental health professional may encounter patients who complain of a low mood and who may have been prescribed antidepressants that seem to give them little help. They may have dysthymia, which is a depressive illness in which milder but persistent symptoms are experienced, which the patient may have had for a period of years. Because of the relatively mild nature of the depression, the patient may have been prescribed low doses of antidepressants, which produce little effect. As a result, such patients may be less compliant if further antidepressant therapy is prescribed because they consider that the treatment does them little good. They may do better with psychotherapy (Stimmel, 1996), but can benefit from antidepressants if they receive similar dosages to those given to patients with major depression. Dysthymia is more common in women than men. Some patients suffer from a combination of dysthymia and major depression.

PATHOPHYSIOLOGICAL CHANGES ASSOCIATED WITH DEPRESSION

The development of non-invasive techniques of brain imaging such as positron emission tomography (PET) has enabled neurophysiologists to develop a better understanding of the living brain. Depressed people have been demonstrated to have reduced blood flow and reduced activity in the frontal temporal cortex and caudate nucleus (Stimmel, 1996). The affected structures are shown in Figure 3.1.

Specific neurotransmitters govern mood. Understanding of the underlying processes of depressive illness was originally developed through observation of the mental effects of amphetamines in the 1930s and during treatment for hypertension by the administration of reserpine in the 1950s. Amphetamines, when given to mildly depressed patients, were noted to improve mood.

They were also known to increase the length of time that noradrenaline (norepinephrine) remained in neuronal synapses. The early studies of the relationship between neurotransmitters and depression caused researchers to propose the biogenic amine hypothesis, which implicated depletion of noradrenaline, dopamine or serotonin at synapses within the central nervous system (CNS) as the cause of depression. These findings continue to be valid. Studies of the levels of noradrenaline, its metabolite 3-methoxy-4-hydroxyophenethyleneglycol (MHPG) and an enzyme breaking down dopamine have been found to

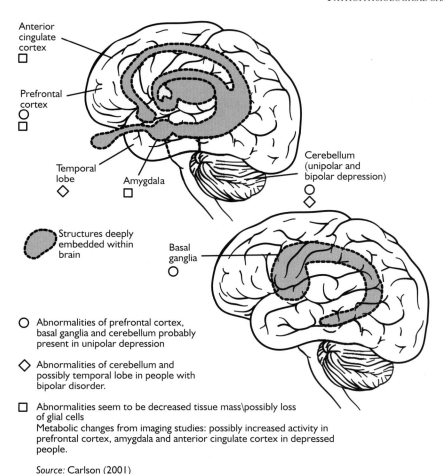

Figure 3.1

Areas of the brain where cerebral activity is altered in depression

Anterior cingulate cortex □

Prefrontal cortex ○ □

Temporal lobe ◇

Amygdala □

Cerebellum (unipolar and bipolar depression) ○ ◇

Structures deeply embedded within brain

Basal ganglia ○

○ Abnormalities of prefrontal cortex, basal ganglia and cerebellum probably present in unipolar depression

◇ Abnormalities of cerebellum and possibly temporal lobe in people with bipolar disorder.

□ Abnormalities seem to be decreased tissue mass\possibly loss of glial cells
Metabolic changes from imaging studies: possibly increased activity in prefrontal cortex, amygdala and anterior cingulate cortex in depressed people.

Source: Carlson (2001)

be altered in the urine and cerebrospinal fluid of depressed patients. Patients who make frequent and determined suicide attempts have been found to have depleted levels in their cerebrospinal fluid of 5-hydroxyindole acetic acid (5-HIAA), a metabolite of serotonin. Some sufferers from major depressive episodes have been demonstrated to have abnormal levels of dopamine and gamma-amino butyric acid (GABA; Judd *et al.*, 1991). Other hypotheses involve the cholinergic system in the brain, with suggestions that acetylcholine levels are increased and out of balance with other neurotransmitter levels in depressed people. Figure 3.2 shows the major neurotransmitter systems that are thought to be imbalanced in depressive illness. In addition, depression produces a stress response, so the hormones of chronic stress (adrenocorticotrophic hormone and cortisol) tend to become elevated.

◀ **Key point**

Although multifactorial in causation, there are biochemical imbalances in the central nervous systems of people with significant depression.

Figure 3.2

Neurotransmitter systems implicated in the aetiology of depression.

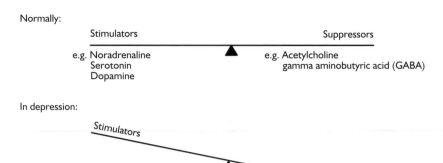

(a)

Local balance between excitatory and inhibitory neurotransmitters is lost within specific synapses

Normally:

Stimulators   Suppressors

e.g. Noradrenaline   e.g. Acetylcholine
Serotonin   gamma aminobutyric acid (GABA)
Dopamine

In depression:

Stimulators

Suppressors

Originally, scientific investigators concentrated on the production, storage and release of neurotransmitters at the presynaptic neurone. Later work has focused upon activities at the postsynaptic neurone, where it is suggested that disordered activity surrounding the binding of the neurotransmitter to the vesicles in the postsynaptic receptors occurs in depressive disorders. It appears that disorders of the neurotransmitters in the opposite direction occur in mania (see below). However, brain scans require the patient to lie still with the head enclosed in a confined space while the investigation takes place and it is clearly easier to scan a relatively immobile person suffering from depression than someone who is hyperactive because of bipolar affective disorder.

Nerve cell receptors can alter their receptivity to adjust to the amounts of neurotransmitter available. A mismatch between the number of neurotransmitter molecules and receptors may be part of the explanation of depressive illness and also its treatment. As antidepressant therapy results in the increase of transmitter molecules present in the synapse, there is an associated decrease in the number of vacant receptors, and this, in general, has the effect of extending the time that free transmitter molecules are present in the synapse

Key point ▶

> Normally, a balance is maintained between the amount of available neurotransmitter substances and the number of active receptors that stimulate the adjacent neurone, thus promoting cerebral activity.

Seasonal affective disorder: depression due to altered biological rhythmicity

A number of people in the northern latitudes find that their moods are adversely affected during the winter months, when there are long hours with poor light levels. The person may complain of feeling 'low', of

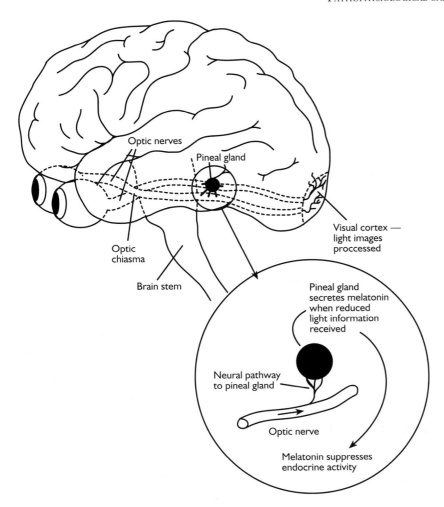

Figure 3.3

The relationship between light and melatonin production

having no energy, may crave carbohydrates and as a result, gain weight (Lewy *et al.*, 1998). Increased amounts of time may be spent asleep. The sufferer from seasonal affective disorder (SAD) seems literally to be in hibernation mode. Experimental work with rats has demonstrated that there exists a neural pathway between the optic nerve tracts and the supraoptic nuclei and the pineal gland (Figure 3.3). Investigation of the pineal gland subsequently found that one of its functions is to produce melatonin, an 'off switch' (or 'hibernation') hormone, which suppresses somatic functioning. Melatonin is therefore implicated as a cause of SAD.

A lack of serotonin and its precursor substance tryptophan has also been implicated in the causation of SAD (Ruhrmann *et al.*, 1998), which may help to explain the appeal of chocolate (which is rich in tryptophan) for some sufferers from SAD. Experimental work has demonstrated that the lowered mood of SAD can be corrected with bright light therapy, which involves the sufferer spending time in proximity to a light source of about 2500–4000 lux, which is about the intensity of light on a bright sunny day (Eastman *et al.*, 1998). The effect of bright light has been found to be enhanced if exposure is combined with a regime of supervised physical exercise (Partonen *et al.*, 1998). Other workers have suggested that the time of day that light therapy is given influences the therapeutic effect, with bright light therapy in the morning having the best effect for most sufferers (Lewy *et al.*,1998). Ruhrmann *et al.* (1998) found that for some patients, the effects of light therapy can be enhanced by the use of fluoxetine, leading them to suggest that serotonin is involved in the pathophysiology of SAD, perhaps by acting as the neurotransmitter in the suprachiasmatic nucleus which functions as the 'body clock' controlling biological rhythmicity.

Key point ▶

> In seasonal affective disorder, it appears that the lack of environmental light causes neurochemical and endocrine changes in the brain, which result in reduced activity levels and lowered mood.

THE MAJOR ANTIDEPRESSANT DRUGS

The group of antidepressants that are now often the first line of antidepressant treatment are the most recently discovered selective serotonin reuptake inhibitors (SSRIs). As will be seen below, the older antidepressant drugs have adverse effects that make them potentially hazardous. For this reason, the SSRI group will be discussed first.

Selective serotonin reuptake inhibitors

As was shown in Figure 3.2, neurotransmitters are secreted at nerve endings, cross the synapse to bind with receptor molecules and are then either broken down by enzymes or pumped back into storage in the synaptic clefts of the axon. Serotonin is returned to storage in readiness for the next action potential and this mechanism is interrupted by SSRIs, thus lengthening the time that serotonin remains active in the synapses. Some SSRIs work primarily at the presynaptic neurone, others at the postsynaptic receptor.

The administration of SSRIs has the additional effect of altering the feedback mechanism by which the postsynaptic receptors upregulate (increase their receptivity) or downregulate (decrease their receptivity) as part of an internal regulatory system. This produces the overall result of increasing neuronal communication as a result of the enhanced concentration of serotonin within the synapses – if a proportion of receptors have 'closed down', then the serotonin remains free and active for longer within the synapse. Thus, SSRIs work by influencing an array of mechanisms that influence nerve transmission within the CNS.

Some clients are less responsive than others to treatment with SSRIs. This is thought to result from individual variations in the regulatory mechanisms at the synapses. Pharmacological research continues to try to develop products that can produce a rapid adjustment of the serotonin concentration at the synapses in the hope of creating a rapid-acting antidepressant.

Selective serotonin reuptake inhibitors have to a large extent become the preferred antidepressant prescribed because of their comparative lack of adverse effects, which make them safer and more acceptable for patients. However, all SSRIs tend to cause nausea, insomnia, anxiety and reduced sexual functioning. In men, delayed ejaculation may occur and women may be unable to reach orgasm. These effects are directly dose-dependent (Stimmel, 1996), so it may be helpful if the prescription can be adjusted to obtain optimal antidepressant effect while minimising the adverse effect. Impaired sexual functioning may initially seem unimportant in view of the fact that the depressed patient probably had a reduced libido as part of the illness, but treatment for major depression may be needed for months. Sustained sexual impairment may produce more problems for the patient and partner if s/he is normally sexually active, and may be a factor in the patient deciding prematurely to stop taking the medication.

A benefit of SSRIs in general is that they appear to be relatively safe when taken in overdose. There is a tendency for manic states to be induced in susceptible subjects and, overall, SSRIs have not been passed as safe to take by pregnant or lactating women, or for use in children. Clients receiving SSRIs may experience **serotonin syndrome** which is thought to be due to an interaction with tryptophan producing restlessness, agitation, gastrointestinal symptoms and hyperthermia.

Selective serotonin reuptake inhibitors, although generally providing safe treatment for some forms of depression, commonly have the effect of interfering with sexual function.

◀ **Key point**

Fluoxetine

This SSRI is probably the best known to the public. It may be prescribed for clients who have depression with or without anxiety and it is useful in enabling individuals to continue with their usual activities because it does not produce sedation. Some users have reported that the use of fluoxetine produces a sense of emotional distancing.

The normal dose for treating depression is 20 mg/day. It is usually presented in capsules containing either 20 mg or 60 mg of fluoxetine but is also available as a syrup containing 20 mg fluoxetine per 5 ml dose. Fluoxetine is also used as treatment for patients with obsessive–compulsive disorder (see Chapter 2) and bulimia nervosa (see Chapter 4). Time is needed for the medication to reach therapeutic levels in the brain, so, in common with other antidepressants, clients need to understand that there will not be an instantaneous improvement when they start taking the drug. Fluoxetine has a long half life of 1–3 days, which extends still more during long-term treatment, so it remains in the plasma for a considerable time after the treatment is stopped. This must be remembered when other treatments are required that may interact with fluoxetine.

Adverse effects and contraindications

Fluoxetine can cause motor restlessness, agitation, anxiety and insomnia. If the client has impaired renal function, fluoxetine is not suitable for long-term treatment because of the risk of toxic accumulation. It is also not suitable for mothers with postnatal depression who are breastfeeding, as the drug is excreted in breast milk, which may cause crying, sleep disturbance, vomiting and watery stools in the infant (Datapharm, 1999). Fluoxetine can produce allergic reactions, so rashes should be noted as the treatment may need to be discontinued. Because the preparation can cause seizures, the mental health professional should carefully monitor its use in clients who suffer from epilepsy. Diabetic clients may find that their blood glucose status becomes destabilised while they are taking fluoxetine. When caring for clients with bipolar conditions, the mental health professional should remember that fluoxetine destabilises lithium levels.

It is possible that fluoxetine may interact with the herb valerian. Yager *et al.* (1999) report the case of a patient prescribed fluoxetine who presented at the mental health clinic with agitation and self-inflicted wounds to his left arm in which he was experiencing abnormal sensations. He was found to have taken some valerian root extract for neck spasms.

Overdoses involving solely fluoxetine seldom cause death, but if a large overdose is taken (around 3000 mg; Datapharm, 2000), nausea and vomiting may occur, as may agitation, restlessness, hypomania and grand mal seizures, which are all consistent with overstimulation of the

---

CASE STUDY 3.1   THOMAS, A CLIENT WITH DEPRESSION

Read this case study and then attempt to answer the questions that follow.

Thomas sought help after his long-term relationship finally foundered. He seems to have entered a world that was entirely grey and in which none of the activities he had previously enjoyed had any meaning. He had previously enjoyed going to clubs and had in the past sometimes taken recreational drugs. Now he had no wish to do anything and simply getting through the day was like walking uphill through treacle. He simply had no energy and the loss of his relationship caused him to feel that he had no personal worth and that there was no point in looking after himself or paying any attention to his personal appearance. He was prescribed fluoxetine. After a while he gradually realised that he was feeling better, in fact he felt quite happy and dissociated from any emotional pain, so he was able to return to his previous social life, where he became the life and soul of the party. Eventually he found a new relationship but now had difficulty because his sex drive seemed to have completely disappeared.

1. What, apart from his failed relationship, might have contributed to Thomas's depression?
2. What factors might have resulted in him deciding to stop the antidepressant therapy?
3. What other antidepressants could have been used that would have avoided this problem?

CNS. There is no specific antidote but activated charcoal is used to bind unabsorbed fluoxetine within the gut.

Sertraline

This preparation is useful in treating depression, with or without anxiety, and is helpful in preventing relapses and recurrence. The usual dose is 50 mg daily: some clients may require a larger dose initially to obtain a therapeutic response. Beneficial effects may become evident after 1 week of treatment, although full activity takes 2-4 weeks to develop. Sertraline is not licensed in the UK for use in children. In susceptible clients, sertraline can induce manic or hypomanic states. It is strongly protein-bound and so absorption may increase markedly when taken with food. Because it influences serotonin uptake without binding to other neuroreceptors, sertraline seems to produce fewer adverse effects than fluoxetine, although clients also taking neuroleptic medication may develop abnormal gait or other movement disorders. It is not considered to produce psychological or physiological dependence but some relatively minor withdrawal effects such as dizziness, headache, anxiety and nausea may occur on ceasing treatment, and medication should be withdrawn slowly when treatment is complete. When sertraline alone is taken in overdose it appears to be relatively safe, although fatalities have occurred when overdosage involves alcohol with or without other drugs.

Paroxetine

The usual antidepressant dose of paroxetine is 20 mg daily and the medication is generally taken once daily in the morning with food. The more common adverse effects include nausea, drowsiness, vomiting and diarrhoea, sweating, tremor and weakness, insomnia, dry mouth and sexual dysfunction. Appetite suppression sometimes occurs. Serotonin syndrome may be caused if paroxetine is taken in conjunction with tryptophan. In overdose, paroxetine is relatively safe. Nausea, vomiting, tremor, dilatation of the pupils, irritability, dry mouth, sweating and drowsiness are among the more common effects. Abrupt discontinuation of treatment with paroxetine may cause withdrawal symptoms of dizziness, headache, anxiety, paraesthesia and nausea. These usually resolve spontaneously. Overdose of paroxetine alone produces drowsiness, coma, rigidity of facial expression, tachycardia, convulsions, vomiting, cyanosis and hyperventilation. Death is rare when the overdose is known not to involve other drugs.

Citalopram

Citalopram is given in a single oral dose of 20 mg daily, although daily doses of up to 60 mg may be given. Because protein binding is relatively low, there are few drug interactions and citalopram is sometimes given, with careful monitoring, to pregnant or lactating women. Citalopram is thought to be one of the most selective of the SSRIs and to have little effect upon noradrenaline (norepinephrine), dopamine or GABA receptors. Adverse effects associated with citalopram are usually mild and of short duration. Nausea, sleepiness, dry mouth, sweating and tremors may be experienced, usually within the first few weeks of treatment. Rapid withdrawal of treatment tends to cause dizziness, paraesthesia, headache, anxiety and nausea. Citalopram is often given to clients who are at increased risk of suicide. The effects of overdose are similar to those of paroxetine poisoning: and may include drowsiness, coma, rigidity of facial expression, tachycardia, convulsions, cyanosis and hyperventilation. Overdose of citalopram alone does not usually cause death.

Dual reuptake inhibitors: serotonin–noradrenaline reuptake inhibitors (SNRIs)

Venlafaxine is a new type of antidepressant that is usually given as 75 mg daily in two divided doses. The preparation is thought to work by potentiating CNS neurotransmitter activity. It inhibits reuptake of serotonin and noradrenaline and additionally has a weak effect upon dopamine reuptake. It may also produce some suppression of the sympathetic beta-receptors. The interactions and contraindications are similar to those for SSRIs. Venlafaxine works in a similar manner to the tricyclic group of antidepressants but lacks their specific adverse actions. Adverse effects of venlafaxine include nausea, headache, sleep disturbances, drowsiness, physical weakness, dry mouth, dizziness, constipation, sweating and feelings of nervousness. Similar symptoms occur on rapid withdrawal of treatment; additionally nervousness and confusion may be experienced. Overdose of venlafaxine may produce alterations to the pulse rate, either tachycardia or bradycardia, and convulsive seizures have been reported. However the overdoses reported tend not to involve venlafaxine in isolation (Datapharm, 2000).

The action of venlafaxine is undergoing comparison with that of the SSRIs and **bupropion** (see below) to establish whether it has a more rapid effect. SNRIs are also being evaluated as agents for the treatment of chronic pain.

Noradrenaline–dopamine reuptake inhibitors (NDRIs)

The drug **bupropion** has an antidepressant effect by increasing the concentration of noradrenaline and dopamine. The product appears to work not only by inhibiting reuptake of these neurotransmitters but also by forming a metabolite that has a more potent effect than the original substance and, in addition, becomes concentrated within the brain. Therefore, the medication that the client takes is in effect a precursor substance, which the body subsequently converts into a more effective agent. For this reason, bupropion is termed a 'prodrug'. A sustained release format is now available. Bupropion is currently used predominantly in the USA. As it does not affect the serotonin system, the sexual dysfunction that accompanies treatment with SSRIs is absent, and it may be useful for patients who are unable to tolerate other adverse effects of SSRIs that occur as a result of serotonin augmentation.

Tricyclic antidepressants

Tricyclics are so called because their biochemical structure is composed of three molecular rings. These products were first developed for the treatment of schizophrenia, for which they were not found to be effective, but the process of clinical testing revealed a therapeutic use for the treatment of depression. These antidepressants are readily lipid soluble and therefore enter the CNS promptly. A significant amount of the drugs are inactivated by hepatic first pass metabolism. Tricyclic antidepressants improve mood by blocking the reuptake of serotonin and noradrenaline and also, to a lesser degree, dopamine.

Tricyclics block cholinergic receptors that are responsive to muscarine (muscarinic receptors) and this causes the unwanted effects of dryness of the mouth, blurring of vision, hesitancy of micturition and constipation. Blockade of H_1 histamine receptors causes weight gain and sedation and alpha-1-adrenergic blockade causes an increased susceptibility to postural hypotension and dizziness.

In common with SSRI antidepressants, care is needed when a client has a tendency to convulsions as tricyclics increase the occurrence of seizures. If the client has a tendency to suffer panic disorders, this may also be exacerbated by taking tricyclic antidepressants. Tricyclics readily react with a range of other medications, so it is important to know if a client is already taking: antihypertensives such as methyldopa; antiparkinsonian drugs; antihistamines; or drugs such as adrenaline (epinephrine), isoprenaline or noradrenaline, which may have been prescribed for conditions such as nasal congestion, cardiovascular problems or bronchial asthma. Older clients may suffer from cardiovascular disorders as well as depression, and for these people tricyclic antidepressants may cause additional problems by destabilising or provoking physical as well as mental ill health. The cardiovascular effects of tricyclic antidepressants make them particularly hazardous when taken in overdose: a 15-day supply is potentially lethal for most patients (Stahl, 1996). Tricyclic antidepressants also potentiate the CNS depressant effect of alcohol.

Imipramine

Imipramine is thought to inhibit the reuptake of noradrenaline and serotonin within the synapses. The normal dose is 25 mg given three times daily. The medication is available as 25 mg tablets, or syrup containing 25 mg in 5 ml. The dose may be gradually increased to control the symptoms, and then reduced to 50–100 mg daily to provide a maintenance dose.

Adverse effects

If a client has a tendency to hypotension, then the blood pressure should be monitored as imipramine can cause postural hypotension, with dizziness or faintness on changing position. Imipramine can cause inhibition of micturition or constipation because of its antagonistic effect on acetylcholine receptors. There is some evidence that long-term treatment with imipramine is associated with increased dental caries (Datapharm, 1999). The use of imipramine has been known to cause a worsening of psychosis in people who suffer from schizophrenia. The effects of alcohol and sedative preparations are enhanced when the client concurrently takes imipramine. Sudden withdrawal of imipramine may provoke nausea, vomiting, abdominal pain, diarrhoea, insomnia, headache, anxiety and nervousness. Overdose produces cardiac arrhythmias, hypotension, cardiac failure and occasionally cardiac arrest. Effects on the CNS include drowsiness, restless, ataxia, restlessness, agitation and then coma. Respiratory depression may occur, also cyanosis, shock fever and reduction or cessation of the urinary output. There is no specific antidote to imipramine poisoning: supportive treatment in a hospital with acute medical facilities is needed.

Nortriptyline

Because of its potential toxicity, patients prescribed nortriptyline require vigilance on the part of the mental health professional. The usual dose for adults is 25 mg three or four times daily. The drug is metabolised by a hepatic enzyme that is reduced in 3–10% of the population; these people are predisposed to toxic effects at normal dosages. For this reason, clients commencing this medication begin by taking a low dose, which is then gradually increased. Elderly patients and adolescents may also have reduced tolerance and may be prescribed a lower dosage, as may patients being treated as outpatients. The therapeutic improvement of mood takes several weeks to become evident, which has obvious implications for the mental health professional caring for clients with suicidal tendencies. If the medication is stopped suddenly, insomnia, irritable mood and increased sweating may occur.

This medication is used as a stimulant of the CNS, and these effects may be problematic for susceptible people. If an epileptic client is prescribed nortriptyline, the mental health professional should watch carefully for convulsive seizures as nortriptyline increases susceptibility to fits (Datapharm, 1999). It is also contraindicated for administration to schizophrenic clients as existing psychosis can be made worse and, if the client is already agitated or hyperactive, these problems may be exacerbated. Similarly, the preparation may provoke the onset of mania in sufferers from bipolar (manic-depressive) disease. Because mental and physical response speeds may be reduced, those receiving nortriptyline are warned against operating hazardous machinery or driving a car. Nortriptyline must not be given concurrently or within 2 weeks of treatment with monoamine oxidase inhibitors (MAOIs) as clients are in danger of developing potentially fatal increases in body temperature (hyperpyrexia) and convulsions. Nortriptyline can destabilise blood glucose levels in diabetic clients, so increased vigilance is needed in this situation.

Rapid withdrawal of treatment may cause feelings of general illness, nausea and headaches. Effects of overdose develop within hours and include visual blurring, confusion, restlessness, dizziness, alterations of body temperature (either fever or hypothermia), agitation, vomiting, dilatation of the pupils, rapid heart rate, convulsive seizures and respiratory depression. Nortriptyline poisoning may respond to intensive resuscitation but it can be lethal.

Amitriptyline

Amitriptyline is given to clients over the age of 16 years in a dose of between 50 and 100 mg at night at the commencement of therapy. The dose is subsequently increased to around 200 mg per day and then reduced to the lowest dose that will maintain the therapeutic response (usually between 50 and 100 mg), given at night. As patients over 65 years of age are susceptible to developing agitation, confusion and postural hypotension when taking this medication, they need careful observation when treatment is commenced and may be prescribed half the normal adult dose as maintenance therapy. In the case of older males with a history of urinary retention, it should be remembered that tricyclics inhibit micturition so they are usually avoided in this client group. Amitriptyline is also best avoided for pregnant and lactating mothers. Infants of mothers who have taken amitriptyline during the last trimester of pregnancy have been reported as suffering from agitation and respiratory depression during the neonatal period. (Datapharm, 1999).

As with other tricyclic antidepressants, abrupt withdrawal after long-term use may cause nausea, malaise and headache. High-dose therapy may cause visual hallucinations, confusion and problems with concentration. Overdosage is associated with drowsiness, rapid irregular pulse, hypothermia, heart failure, hypotension, convulsions and coma.

Dosulepin (dothiepin)

Dosulepin is helpful for treating clients whose depression is associated with anxiety. The initial dose is 75 mg daily, which may be given as a single dose at night or in divided doses during the day. Following commencement of therapy, the dose is increased to perhaps 20–50 mg three times daily or 75–150 mg as a single night-time dose. As with other tricyclic antidepressants, particular care is needed when establishing older clients on the medication, and they may be prescribed half of the normal adult dose. Dosulepin is not recommended for use for children, pregnant or lactating women and is contraindicated for clients suffering from mania. It should be avoided if clients are subject to epileptic seizures. If taken with alcohol, the depressant effects of alcohol upon the CNS are increased. Dosulepin decreases alertness, so an appropriate warning should be given about driving cars or operating heavy machinery. It also produces atropine-like affects, which include dryness of the mouth and difficulty in focussing vision. Constipation and hesitation of micturition may occur during stabilisation on dosulepin treatment.

Withdrawal symptoms may include sweating, insomnia and irritability. If dosulepin is taken in overdose the symptoms include mental excitement and visual hallucinations, dryness of the mouth, ataxia, convulsions, coma, dilatation of the pupils, rapid irregular pulse, hypotension and respiratory depression.

| **CASE STUDY 3.2** | **MAXINE, A CLIENT WHO HAS BEEN PRESCRIBED A TRICYCLIC ANTIDEPRESSANT** |

Read this case study and then attempt to answer the questions that follow.

'Oh, I've got so much to do and no energy to do it!' In fact, Maxine had the washing up to do, a letter to write to the bank to cancel a standing order, and a few phone calls to make. These tasks left Maxine feeling quite weighed down: they seemed to be haunting her every waking minute. Every morning she was waking early and then lay terrified about the challenges imposed by the day ahead, and whether today would be the day when she was finally found out as being incompetent – the thoughts in her brain seemed to have been replaced by volumes of cotton wool. Life had become a grey fog. Maxine was prescribed a tricyclic antidepressant.

1. Why would Maxine find that she did not immediately feel better from taking the antidepressant?
2. What factor would have influenced the choice of Maxine's antidepressant?
3. Maxine found that she was not easily able to concentrate when she tried to read the newspaper. She also found after a period of time that she was putting on weight. What is the reason for these effects?

Monoamine oxidase inhibitors

This group of antidepressants was discovered in the early 1950s during a search for products that would be effective against tuberculosis. Iproniazid, which inhibits synaptic enzymes, was noticed to improve the mood of severely depressed patients and from this observation developed a mass of clinical trials. MAOIs tend nowadays to be used for clients who do not respond to other antidepressants. Their use is restricted by their reactivity with certain foodstuffs and other medications and the resultant hazards for clients.

Monoamine oxidase inhibitors work by blocking the breakdown of the CNS stimulatory neurotransmitters adrenaline, noradrenaline and dopamine. Following commencement of therapy, between 2 and 4 weeks are required for the maximum therapeutic effect to be achieved. MAOIs can cause agitation, insomnia and restlessness and manic states can be induced in clients with bipolar disease. Because MAOIs produce insomnia, the medication must be taken well before the client's sleep time, so the last dose of the day is usually timed before 6pm to avoid disturbance of sleep. Unlike the tricyclic antidepressants, MAOIs do not induce convulsive seizures, so they can be useful for people with epilepsy. Some side-effects, such as postural hypotension, delayed ejaculation, failure to achieve orgasm, weight gain and oedema occur fairly commonly. In addition to being prescribed multiple drugs (polypharmacy) with the added increased risk of interactions with

MAOIs, older clients may suffer from postural hypotension, which may limit the use of MAOIs in this group of people. Because of the hazard of blood pressure disturbances, MAOIs are not recommended in those with a history of transient ischaemic attack or stroke. If a client has reason to need a local anaesthetic, it is important that preparations containing adrenaline (epinephrine) are avoided because of the danger of provoking hypertension. Cardiovascular effects, coma and disordered temperature control make significant overdosage of MAOIs hazardous.

There are two forms of monoamine oxidase, MAO A and MAO B. MAO A breaks down serotonin and noradrenaline. In addition to mood preservation, noradrenaline exerts a profound effect upon blood pressure, so the effects of MAO A antidepressants are sometimes complicated by hypotension. The B form of MAO can produce neurotoxins by converting precursor substances into active forms, which are then thought to produce neurodegenerative states. MAO B inhibitors, therefore, have potential use for the treatment of conditions such as Parkinson's disease. Pharmacological advances have meant that selective MAO A or B inhibitors can now be made and also that the action of the agents can be made reversible. Reversible MAO A (RIMA) antidepressants are now available, which makes treatment with this group of antidepressants safer and reduces the need for the client to avoid tyramine-rich foods. RIMA antidepressants are also valuable for the treatment of clients suffering from panic disorder and social phobia (see Chapter 2).

A potentially fatal interaction

Unfortunately, MAOIs inhibit the metabolism of tyramine within the liver and gastrointestinal tract. If food rich in tyramine (such as mature cheese, yogurt, yeast extracts, broad beans, sauerkraut and dried sausage such as pepperoni or salami) is eaten, the excessive tyramine may cause a large-scale release of noradrenaline and a consequent dramatic rise in the blood pressure that, in extreme cases, may be fatal. Certain drugs such as ephedrine, amphetamines, levodopa and SSRIs interact with MAOIs to cause a similar effect.

Phenelzine

Phenelzine has been found to be useful for clients who have mixed anxiety and depression, which may also be complicated by phobias and morbid fears related to their physical health. One 15 mg tablet three times daily is usually given and effects are often observed within a week. If effects are not seen within 2 weeks, the dose is usually increased to a maximum of 15 mg four times daily. Once stabilised, the client may be prescribed a maintenance dose of 15 mg on alternate days. Phenelzine is not recommended for use in children or pregnant or lactating women.

The drug should be withdrawn gradually at the end of treatment to avoid the risk of the client experiencing nightmares, agitation or hallucinations. Signs and symptoms of overdose tend to develop between 12–

48 hours after ingestion. Drowsiness, dizziness, hyperactivity and irritation, faintness, headaches and hallucinations may occur. The pulse may become rapid and irregular and shock may develop. If a large overdose is taken, the client may be euphoric or hypomanic and then sink into coma with respiratory depression and hyperpyrexia. Early recognition and supportive medical treatment is important, as large overdoses may be lethal.

Tranylcypromine

This is another product used for significant depressive episodes that are accompanied by phobic symptoms or are resistant to treatment with other agents. The drug is licensed for treatment of adults only and is given in initial doses of 10 mg orally twice a day for a week, following which an additional 5 mg is given at midday. Once the client's symptoms come under control, a maintenance dose of 10 mg a day is continued. Tranylcypromine may be given, if needed, in conjunction with a tranquilliser, but it is important to ascertain that the client does not have a history of dependence upon drugs or alcohol, as dependence and tolerance of high doses of tranylcypromine sometimes occurs.

Adverse effects include insomnia, headache, drowsiness, weakness and restlessness, and hypomania may be produced in susceptible clients. Overdosage produces exaggerated versions of the adverse effects. Tremor, convulsions and hyperpyrexia may develop gradually, along with hypotension.

Moclobemide

This agent is used for major depressive episodes, particularly associated with socially induced phobias. It must be given with care (and perhaps, benzodiazepine sedation) when the client is agitated. The tablets are taken following meals. An initial dose of 300 mg daily in divided doses is followed by a maintenance dose of 150 mg when the symptoms are controlled. No special restrictions are required for older clients. The preparation is not licensed for use on children and it is not certain that it is completely safe for use by pregnant or lactating women. It should not be given to clients suffering from acute confusional states or Parkin-son's disease, and it cannot be given with selegiline. If taken in conjunction with some cough remedies, there may be adverse CNS effects, as moclobemide interacts with dextromethorphan, which is a constituent of certain proprietary cough medicines. In comparison with other MAOIs, moclobemide produces less difficulty related to inter-action with tyramine-rich foods, so dietary restriction is usually less crucial with this product, although an unknown (but small) proportion of the population is particularly sensitive, so as a rule, clients are advised to avoid such foods (see above).

Adverse effects include sleep disturbances, anxiety and agitation, restlessness, irritability, dizziness, dry mouth, paraesthesia, visual distur-bances, nausea and vomiting, diarrhoea and constipation. Transient confusional states sometimes occur. Signs of overdosage include

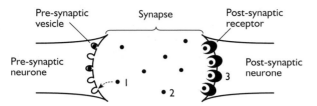

Figure 3.4

Mode of action of antidepressant drugs

Drugs may

(1) Inhibit reuptake of transmitter into synaptic vesicles of pre-synaptic neurone.
(2) Inhibit release of transmitter from post-synaptic receptors.
(3) Influence down-regulation of post synaptic receptors

SSRIs increase the concentration of serotonin in the synapses.

SARIs (serotonin-2 antagonists/reuptake inhibitors) inhibit return of serotonin to pre-synaptic vesicles.

Dual Reuptake Inhibitors influence more than 1 transmitter system, e.g.
Serotonin and noradrenaline (SNRIs)
Noradrenaline and dopamine (NDRIs)

Tetracyclics inhibit noradrenaline uptake
Tricyclics inhibit return of noradrenaline and serotonin to presynaptic vesicles.

MAOIs increase secretion and inhibit breakdown of noradrenaline and serotonin at synapses.

agitation and aggressiveness. If the overdose involves a combination of other agents affecting the CNS, there is an increased risk of death. Fig. 3.4 summarises the mode of action of antidepressant drugs.

Changing antidepressant medication

Because of the potentially fatal danger of hyperthermia, muscular rigidity, extreme agitation, delirium, coma and loss of autonomic nervous system control when SSRIs and MAOIs are in the system concurrently, it is important that health professionals prescribing changes in medication allow around 14 days 'washout time' between discontinuing MAOIs and commencing fluoxetine. If MAOIs are to be used following fluoxetine, it may be necessary to wait for a minimum of 5 weeks between the two treatments. Similarly, if a client's prescription is being changed between an MAOI and a tricyclic antidepressant, sufficient time must elapse for the original medication to be excreted in order to avoid severe hypertension, hyperpyrexia, agitation, neuromuscular seizures, delirium and coma.

Phenylpiperazines

This group of substances act via blockade of serotonin-2 receptors and inhibition of the reuptake of serotonin, so they are classified as serotonin-2-antagonist/reuptake inhibitors, abbreviated to SARIs.

Trazodone

This product was developed during the search for products that would supersede the tricyclic family of antidepressants. Trazodone has both antidepressant and anxiolytic properties and works by influencing the metabolism of serotonin by blocking the serotonin-2 receptors. There is also a very weak inhibition of noradrenaline uptake from the synapses.

Trazodone is given in a starting dose of 150 mg a day, either after meals or as a single dose before sleeping. If necessary, the dose may be increased to 300 mg per day taken in divided doses. Because of the sedative effect, clients are advised to avoid operating hazardous machinery. Trazodone interacts with phenytoin, producing raised levels of this, which must be remembered if it is prescribed for clients who are being treated concurrently for epilepsy. Because of the lack of anticholinergic activity, trazodone spares clients the dryness of mouth that can be a problem for those treated with tricyclic antidepressants. In some men, use of this product may cause the side-effect of priapism – prolonged, painful penile erection, which, if untreated, can ultimately cause vascular damage to the penis. Reversal of priapism is achieved by injecting an alpha-adrenergic agonist into the penis.

Overdosage with trazodone tends to produce drowsiness, dizziness and vomiting, and hypotension may develop.

Nefazodone

Nefazodone is a phenylpiperazine antidepressant that does not impair sexual function. It blocks type 2 serotonin receptors and so impedes serotonin reuptake. It seems to have relatively few adverse effects and causes less sedation than trazodone, which is thought to be because there is a weaker blockade of the histamine receptors. The usual adult dose is 200 mg twice daily. The clinical effects become evident within a week, but full effectiveness is not achieved for several weeks. Nefazodone is not as yet known to be safe for use by pregnant or lactating women or by children.

The SARI group of antidepressants works predominantly upon the serotonin-2 (5-HT$_2$) receptors (5-HT, or 5-hydroxytryptamine, is the biochemical name for serotonin). Adverse actions may result: stimulation of the serotonin-2 receptors in the forebrain can result in anxiety or agitation; stimulation of the same receptors in the spinal cord may produce sexual dysfunction. In practice, however, the SARI group does seem to be more tolerable to some clients. Within the SARI group, trazodone and nefazodone, although chemically related, affect slightly different mechanisms. For example, nefazodone has less antihistamine activity than trazodone and so produces less unwanted sedation. Nefazodone is less associated with postural hypotension and priapism than trazodone. These considerations will influence the choice of prescription for a given client. Generally, nefazodone produces few adverse effects, although weakness, dry mouth, nausea and constipation may occur. These symptoms tend to subside as the dose is adjusted.

Overdoses of nefazodone seem to be relatively rare. Drowsiness and vomiting occur most commonly, although enhanced forms of the documented adverse reactions may also be experienced.

Tetracyclic antidepressants

Maprotiline
Maprotiline has properties that are similar to those of the tricyclic antidepressants, although it is chemically unrelated to them. It improves mood because it is a powerful and specific inhibitor of the reuptake of noradrenaline. It is used for moderate or severe episodes of depression. An initial dose of 75 mg daily is augmented gradually as necessary to a maximum of 150 mg. When the symptoms are controlled, which may take 2–3 weeks, the lowest dose that maintains the improved state is used to continue treatment. The agent is contraindicated for people with epilepsy or another tendency to convulsive seizures. Most adverse reactions are mild and short-lived.

Rapid withdrawal of treatment may produce nausea, vomiting, abdominal pain and diarrhoea. Acute withdrawal can also cause nervousness, headache, nervousness, anxiety and return of the pre-existing depression. Overdose may cause restlessness and agitation, ataxia drowsiness and convulsions and coma. The pulse may become rapid and irregular and respiratory depression may develop. Fever, sweating and reduction or cessation of the urinary output may occur.

Venlafaxine
This agent is a serotonin and noradrenaline reuptake inhibitor used for major depressive episodes. A daily dose of 75 mg is given in two divided doses of 35.5 mg with food. This may be increased to 75 mg daily if needed for severely depressed patients. No special precautions need to be taken for elderly patients who have normal kidney function, but the agent is not known to be safe for the treatment of pregnant or lactating women or children. Several months of treatment are needed for clients suffering from severe depression.

The dosage needs to be tapered on discontinuation of treatment as withdrawal symptoms may otherwise be produced. These include fatigue, headache, nausea and vomiting, dizziness, dry mouth, insomnia, nervousness and confusion, sweating, paraesthesia and vertigo. Overdosage may produce seizures and disturbances of the pulse, either tachycardia or bradycardia. The effects are exacerbated if alcohol has been taken in addition.

L-tryptophan

Tryptophan is an amino acid precursor of serotonin. Administration of tryptophan alone failed to achieve impressive alterations to depressed mood, but the effects were improved when tryptophan was experimentally added to clomipramine. Tryptophan lack has been suggested as a causation of major depressive episodes in addition to seasonal affective disorder (see below).

L-tryptophan is used for patients who suffer from severe disabling depressive illness that is not amenable to treatment with the standard armament of antidepressive drugs. It is prescribed to augment more conventional products and is currently subject to evaluation. Two 500 mg tablets three times a day are usually given. L-tryptophan must not be given in conjunction with MAOIs and sexual disinhibition may occur if it is given in conjunction with phenothiazines or benzodiazepines. There also seems to be an interaction with fluoxetine when prescribed in high doses: the combination can produce agitation, exacerbations of obsessive–compulsive disorder, insomnia, aggression, headaches and other manifestations of serotonin syndrome. When given alone, L-tryptophan may produce drowsiness or slight nausea (Fugh-Berman and Cott, 1999). L-tryptophan can also produce headache and feelings of lightheadedness. Overdosage may cause drowsiness and vomiting.

Alternative remedies

An American review of complementary and alternative medications used for self-treatment of depressive illness (Fugh-Berman and Cott, 1999) identified a range of herbal and other products that are employed, often with no consultation with either a medical or a complementary practitioner.

St John's wort (*Hypericum perforatum*) has been evaluated in comparison with tricyclic antidepressants and was found to perform in a comparable manner. There were fewer reports of adverse effects associated with taking the herbal remedy in comparison with tricyclics, but tricyclics appeared to have a slight advantage in respect of reduction of depressive symptoms. Laboratory tests have demonstrated that St John's wort has a MAOI effect and there is some suggestion that it interacts with serotonin, noradrenaline and dopamine as well as the inhibitory transmitter GABA. St John's wort seems to produce mild adverse effects: fatigue, mild gastrointestinal symptoms and, in fair skinned people, mild temporary photosensitisation. There is a report of undue sedation in a woman who switched between St John's wort and paroxetine (Gordon, 1998). Animal studies have identified no adverse effect upon fertility and reproduction associated with St John's wort.

There is evidence to suggest that depression may be associated with **folic acid** deficiency, and this may relate particularly to elderly people. A link has been made between a lack of dietary folate and the possession of a melancholic disposition! Deficiency of **vitamin B$_{12}$** has also been associated with depression. The altered metabolism of monoamines in depression has been linked with lack of tetrahydrobiopterin, a substance that is necessary for the synthesis of serotonin and dopamine. Reduced synthesis of *S*-adenosyl-methionine (**SAMe**), a chemical that acts as a donor of methyl compounds, has been demonstrated in deficiency of folate and vitamin B_{12}. Administration of SAMe has been observed to be associated with antidepressant effects and, in common with the major antidepressants, also to be associated with the development of mania in people with bipolar affective illness.

In view of the reactivity of a number of the groups of antidepressant drugs, it is to be hoped that other medication was not being taken concurrently!

Phenylalanine and **tyrosine** are amino acids that are precursors of catecholamines. An artificial variant of tyrosine, which is thought to compete with naturally produced tyrosine resulting in depletion of dopamine and noradrenaline, was observed to be associated with a return of low mood in previously depressed subjects.

Omega-3 fatty acids such as arachidonic acid are vital for the formation of the phospholipid cell membrane. Lack of omega-3 fatty acids has been suggested to be a significant contributor to depression as well as other mental and neurological illnesses. **Cholesterol-reducing drugs** used to treat atheromatous blood vessel disease have been linked with serotonin depletion and increased incidence of suicide.

Currently electroconvulsive therapy (ECT) remains the only rapidly acting treatment for severe depression. Although it has been used for decades, the actual mechanism by which it is effective remains unclear. The current explanation is that the seizure induced by the electric current mobilises neurotransmitters into the synapses. Experimental work suggests that the regulation of the neuroreceptors may also be altered to achieve the antidepressant effect. The social acceptability of ECT and the amnesic effect upon the client mean that the search continues to find a pharmacological product that is capable of replacing ECT as a treatment for major depression.

Box 3.1

Electroconvulsive therapy as treatment for depression

BIPOLAR AFFECTIVE DISORDER

Bipolar affective disorder, as its name suggests, involves the sufferer in a series of oscillating mood swings from the downheartedness of depression to the elation and energy of mania. It can be easily appreciated that the state of mania may be perceived as more pleasant (if in some ways less safe!) than that of depression. During the period of elation, the individual feels charged with energy, invincible, perhaps superhuman. Unfortunately, insight may be lost and judgmental errors may generate an epidemic of problems for the sufferer as the manic phase subsides or, before that, for the partner, family or friends trying to help to deal with the excesses that have resulted from the patient's unrealistic, manic behaviour. The sufferer from bipolar affective disorder may oscillate between mania and major depression, interspersed with periods of normal mood or hypomania – a less extreme state of mental hyperactivity. At times, the symptoms of mania and depression may be present simultaneously.

If a person suffers from four or more episodes of mania or depression in a year, they are described as having a rapid-cycling form of the condition. Bipolar disease is classified into two forms, bipolar I disorder in which there are major episodes of depression and mania and bipolar II disorder in which major depression is intermixed with hypomanic episodes.

CASE STUDY 3.3 JASON, A CLIENT WITH BIPOLAR DISORDER

Read this case study and then attempt to answer the questions that follow.

Jason had 'arrived'. He was a rock star of note and would be performing at Wembley in a week's time. He needed to get his stage clothes ready for this and had just had himself measured for a sequinned jump suit and had used his credit card to purchase some snakeskin biker boots at a cost of £800 to complete the outfit. The world smiled upon him, and he was next going to look for a car to suit his persona. He gave the last money he had in his pocket (a £20 note) to one of his fans, a young man in khaki sitting on the pavement with a dog on a string. He needed to sort out the bank, as the cash dispenser had declined to give him any more money that day – obviously the bank had a cash flow problem and needed some financial advice from him. He'd see to that once the car was organised. He felt fantastic – no need for recreational drugs for him! He had completely forgotten ever feeling 'low'.

1. What are likely to be the problems in establishing appropriate pharmacological control of Jason's condition?
2. What is the significance of the mention of recreational drugs in Jason's case?
3. What pharmacological treatment may be prescribed for Jason?

A less extreme form of bipolar disease involves long-term mood disturbance in which mood elevation and depression interrupt short periods of normal mood. This condition, called cyclothymia, is not associated with psychotic episodes and may not cause the individual to seek health care. Sometimes it is seen in relatives of people known to be suffering from established bipolar disease.

It has been seen earlier that the neurotransmitters noradrenaline, serotonin and dopamine become depleted in depression. Therefore it is logical that mania might be the result of the opposite imbalance of neurotransmitters. There is a genetic predisposition to bipolar affective disorders: Stimmel (1996) suggests that between 60% and 65% of sufferers from bipolar disorder have a family member who is similarly affected.

Bipolar affective disorder has been associated with disturbance of the natural biological rhythms. Normal rhythmicity is the result of interaction between the suprachiasmic nuclei and the pineal gland at the base of the brain (see seasonal affective disorder, above, and Chapter 2). The centres for rhythmicity are influenced by environmental light levels as well as social and psychological factors. Some of the biological rhythms are organised to recur around a daily cycle and are termed **circadian rhythms**. In fact, normal circadian rhythms are organised around a 25-hour cycle (Case and Waterhouse, 1994) It has been observed that people with mania have circadian rhythms that cycle more frequently than the normal and, interestingly, antimania drugs such as lithium produce a corrective lengthening in the circadian cycle.

In bipolar disorder, there is disturbance of neural cell function, neuro-transmitter levels and loss of some of the normal biological rhythms.

Medication used to control bipolar disorder

Lithium

Lithium is given for episodes of acute mania. The exact way in which it works remains obscure: it has been suggested that second-messenger systems or G-proteins that activate cell function after the nerve cell receptors are activated may be inhibited. Lithium is thought to reduce the cycles of mood change and the extreme elevations or depressions of mood. From commencement of treatment about 7–10 days are required before therapeutic plasma levels are attained. During this time, antipsychotics are needed to control the client: the dose of these is tapered off once therapeutic lithium levels have been achieved. Lithium treatment should result in an improvement of the bipolar symptoms within a further 2 weeks. Sudden discontinuation of lithium treatment may result in a relapse due to a rebound phenomenon.

Lithium is taken up unevenly in the tissues, appearing in greater concentration in the brain, thyroid and saliva. It is eliminated via the kidneys and removed from the body more slowly in older clients. Lithium has a narrow therapeutic margin: there is little leeway between a therapeutic and a toxic level. For this reason, patients receiving this treatment need to have regular blood specimens taken for estimation of the plasma lithium level – this should be maintained between 0.6 and 0.8 mEq/litre. Levels of more than 1.5 mEq/litre produce toxic effects. Typically, a client may be started on a dose of 300 mg three times daily and the dose is then subsequently titrated to achieve therapeutic plasma levels, so the mental health professional should expect to be helping the client to take varying doses until a steady-state drug level is achieved. Clients who lack insight and who tend to cycle into repeated bipolar episodes may be given lithium treatment as prophylaxis.

Adverse effects

Before lithium therapy is commenced, the client should be screened for cardiovascular, renal and endocrine function. When a therapeutic dose is achieved, the most common adverse effects experienced by clients include thirst and increased micturition, which occurs because lithium blocks the effect of antidiuretic hormone. There may also be an increase in body weight, confusion and slowness of intellect. At therapeutic doses, clients may experience nausea, diarrhoea, muscular weakness and may have a fine tremor of the hands. If lithium toxicity develops, these adverse effects become more pronounced. Long-term lithium therapy is associated with renal damage, so clients receiving prolonged treatment need to have their renal function monitored through estimation of blood urea, creatinine and electrolytes. Monitoring of the specific gravity of the urine is important because the toxic effects result in the impairment of renal concentration of urine, which will result in the passage of copious dilute urine. Lithium toxicity also causes impaired thyroid function. The client may develop a goitre, with a swelling in the front of the neck, and, because lithium inhibits production of thyroxine, may become hypothyroid (see Chapter 8).

Clients receiving long-term lithium treatment frequently gain weight. In part, this may be a result of extra calories being consumed in drinks because of the thirst that lithium therapy produces. The treatment can also cause a worsening of pre-existing skin conditions such as dermatitis, acne or psoriasis, so the mental health professional should note if the client complains of skin rashes. Female clients taking lithium should avoid becoming pregnant while receiving treatment as the drug causes malformation of the fetus if taken in the first 12 weeks of pregnancy. Although lithium may be taken later in pregnancy, it should be gradually discontinued prior to the birth as otherwise toxicity may occur as a result of the fluid shifts that occur during labour and delivery. Overdose causes enhanced versions of the symptoms of lithium toxicity. Severe overdoses may produce seizures, coma and death.

As a result of the many adverse effects of lithium, research continues to create improved mood-stabilising drugs, for instance by altering the action of G-proteins and second-messenger systems (see Chapter 1).

Carbamazepine

Although this agent is more commonly used as an anticonvulsive agent, carbamazepine may be used for prophylactic treatment of manic-depressive psychosis. It is usually given orally in two or three divided doses giving a total dosage of 400–600 mg daily. Carbamazepine is chemically related to MAOIs, so should not be given in combination with these agents. At the commencement of treatment, carbamazepine may produce symptoms including dizziness, ataxia, fatigue and drowsiness, diplopia, nausea and vomiting. If taken in overdose, the CNS and cardiorespiratory system are affected. The client may be drowsy, disorientated, agitated or disoriented with hallucinations, and may subsequently become comatose. Respiratory depression may develop, also a rapid irregular pulse and hypo- or hypertension. Reduction of the urinary output may also occur.

Other agents

The treatment of bipolar affective disorder is complex. The patient's mood may be stabilised by using agents such as lithium or **sodium valproate**. Long-term use of such medication has been found in some cases to be associated with rapid cycling between depression and mania. For the effects of overdose of sodium valproate, see Chapter 8. Problems can also be caused by adverse effects such as tardive dyskinesia and extrapyramidal symptoms (Ghaemi *et al.*, 1999). Ghaemi *et al.* suggest that the incidence of these adverse effects is reduced if the patient who is resistant to treatment is treated with atypical antipsychotic drugs such as **clozapine,** which they suggest has a specific action as a mood stabiliser. Patients receiving clozapine need to have their white blood cell counts monitored during the first 6 months of treatment because of the risk of increased susceptibility to infection due to agranulocytosis.

Risperidone is associated with a reduced risk of agranulocytosis and tardive dyskinesia and fewer anticholinergic side-effects such as dryness of the mouth and blurring of vision. Risperidone therapy also appears to be advantageous in that it does not worsen mood. **Olanzapine** is another antipsychotic agent that appears to be potentially useful for the short-term treatment of mania, as it has short-term antimanic effects, but may not be useful as prophylactic treatment. In summary, some clients who are difficult to treat pharmaceutically with conventional antimania drugs may be helped by taking products known primarily for their anticonvulsive or antipsychotic affects. Such treatment at present is being evaluated in clinical trials.

◀ *Key point*

Bipolar affective disorder presents a challenge to health professionals when the client's condition cycles rapidly between extremes of behaviour. The hazards of lithium therapy have led to continued research into appropriate pharmacological treatment, and some antipsychotic compounds offer promising alternatives.

Box 3.2

Clinical signs of mania

Identifiable periods during which the mood is markedly altered. Rapid mood swings may be noted. For a period of at least a week, at least three of the following are present:

- Reduced need for sleep
- Greatly increased self esteem or feelings of grandeur
- Talking more than usual
- Flight of ideas, sense of racing thoughts
- Easily distracted
- Psychomotor agitation
- Engagement in 'risky' pleasurable experiences
- Impaired social or occupational judgement
- Hallucinations or delusions
- Needs hospitalisation to protect from harm to self or others

Hypomania is characterised by similar features without impaired social or occupational performance. The symptoms last at least four days. Psychosis is not present.

SUMMARY

The disorders of affect may in some cases be viewed as an exaggerated form of normal personality traits. Depression is caused by a multitude of factors but there is an underlying biochemical abnormality responsible for the client's symptoms. This is also the case in bipolar illness. Advances in understanding the neurobiological basis of depression have led to the development of an array of new antidepressant drugs that are generally more acceptable in their relative lack of adverse effects. They are also generally safer than the older forms of antidepressant if taken in overdose. Clients with bipolar disease present a challenge to mental health professionals because the effects are the result of rapid cycling between opposing neurobiological mechanisms.

REFERENCES AND FURTHER READING

Case, R.M. and Waterhouse, J. (1994) *Human Physiology: Age, Stress and the Environment*. Oxford University Press, Oxford.

Datapharm (1999) *ABPI Compendium of Data Sheets*. Datapharm Communications, London.

Datapharm (2000) *ABPI Compendium of Data Sheets*. Datapharm Communications, London.

Eastman, C.I., Young, M.A. Fogg, L.F. *et al.* (1998) Bright light treatment of winter depression: a placebo controlled trial. *Archives of General Psychiatry*, **55**, 883–889.

Fugh-Berman, A. and Cott, J.M. (1999) Dietary supplements and natural products as psychotherapeutic agents. *Psychosomatic Medicine*, **81**, 712–737.

Ghaemi, S., Nassir, M.D. and Goodwin, F.K. (1999) Use of atypical antipsychotic agents in bipolar and schizoaffective disorders: review of the empirical literature. *Journal of Clinical Pharmacology*, **18**, 354–361.

Gordon, J.B. (1998) SSRIs and St John's wort: possible toxicity? *American Family Physician*, **57**, 953.

Judd, L.L. (1991) In: *Harrison's Principles of Internal Medicine*, (eds J.D. Wilson, E. Braunwald, K.J. Isselbacher *et al.*) McGraw Hill, New York.

Lewy, A.J., Bauer, V.K., Cutler, N.L. *et al.* (1998) Morning vs evening light treatment of patients with winter depression. *Archives of General Psychiatry*, **55**, 890–896.

Malt, U.F., Robak, O.H., Madsbu, H.-P. *et al.* (1999) The Norwegian naturalistic treatment study of depression in general practice (NORDEP)-1: randomised double blind study. *British Medical Journal*, **318**, 1180–1184.

Partonen, T., Leppamaki, S., Hurme, J. and Lonnqvist, J. (1998) Randomised trial of physical exercise alone or combined with bright light on mood and health-related quality of life. *Psychological Medicine*, **28**, 1359–1364.

Rippere, V. and Williams, R. (1985) *Wounded Healers: Mental Health Workers' Experiences of Depression*. John Wiley & Sons, Chichester.

Ruhrmann, S., Kasper, S., Hawellek, B. *et al.* (1998) Effects of fluoxetine in the treatment of seasonal affective disorder. *Psychological Medicine*, **28**, 923–933.

Shaw, CM., Creed, F., Tomenson, B *et al.* (1999) Prevalence of anxiety and depressive illness and help-seeking behaviour in African Caribbeans and white Europeans: two phase general population survey. *British Medical Journal*, **318**, 302–305.

Stahl, S.M. (1996) *Essential Psychopharmacology : Neuroscientific Basis and Practical Applications*. Cambridge University Press, Cambridge.

Stimmel, G.L. (1996) Mood disorders. In: *Textbook of Therapeutics* (eds E.T. Herfindal and D.R. Gourley). Williams & Wilkins, Baltimore, MD.

Yager, J., Siegfried, S.L. and DiMatteo, T.L. (1999) Use of alternative remedies by psychiatric patients: illustrative vignettes and a discussion of the issues. *American Journal of Psychiatry*, **156**, 1432–1438.

Websites

Depression: http://www.focusondepression.com/script/Main/hp.asp
Bipolar disease: http://health.yahoo.com/health/dc001528/0.html

SELF-TEST QUESTIONS

Identify the correct answer in the following statements. For each, some, all or no options may be correct.

1. Which of the following statements correctly describe a major depressive illness?
   a. apathy, delusions, anhedonia, low self-esteem
   b. agitation, guilt, lack of enthusiasm, impaired cognition
   c. hallucinations, altered life circumstances, fatigue, poor concentration
   d. indecisiveness, anhedonia, weight change, altered sleep
2. A depressed client has psychomotor retardation. This is likely to be due to:
   a. the antidepressant treatment
   b. bipolar disease
   c. interactions between the antidepressant and other medication
   d. benzodiazepines
3. Dysthymic clients:
   a. may not be identified as having a depressive illness
   b. are often helped by psychotherapy
   c. often discontinue antidepressant treatment prematurely
   d. are more commonly male than female
4. Which of the following combination of neurotransmitters may depleted in depression?
   a. acetylcholine, noradrenaline (norepinephrine), tryptophan, serotonin (5-HT)
   b. adrenaline (epinephrine), dopamine, serotonin, melatonin
   c. gamma-aminobutyric acid, L-tryptophan, arginine, histamine
   d. serotonin, dopamine, noradrenaline, benzodiazepine
5. Which of the following statements about depression is correct?
   a. binding of neurotransmitters to postsynaptic receptors is impaired
   b. storage in the presynaptic cleft is excessive
   c. there are fewer postsynaptic receptors
   d. neural transmission is reduced
6. Which of these statements about selective serotonin reuptake inhibitors are correct?
   a. they tend to cause anxiety

      b.   sleep disturbances may be produced

      c.   gastrointestinal symptoms may occur

      d.   they are safe for use by pregnant women

7.   Serotonin–noradrenaline reuptake inhibitors such as venlafaxine

      a.   act upon the histamine receptor system

      b.   cause drying of the mouth and visual disturbances

      c.   inhibit beta-adrenergic receptors

      d.   influence dopamine, serotonin (5-HT) and noradrenaline (norepinephrine) systems

8.   Tricyclic antidepressants have which of the following properties?

      a.   can cause constipation

      b.   may cause postural hypotension

      c.   tend to interact with other medication

      d.   are slowly taken up in the CNS

9.   Mono-amine oxidase inhibitors:

      a.   are now available in reversible formats

      b.   can cause hypotension

      c.   can cause hypertension

      d.   can provoke manic symptoms

10. Bipolar affective disease:

      a.   can run in families

      b.   disrupts normal biological rhythms

      c.   is exacerbated by sudden cessation of lithium treatment

      d.   can be treated with carbamazepine.

DISORDERS OF EATING AND SLEEPING

4

INTRODUCTION

We eat to provide our bodies with fuel to power the creation of adenosine triphosphate (ATP), the energy molecule that is constructed in the mitochondria of the cells. The ATP is then used as the source of chemical energy, which is used for a multitude of purposes, from synthesis of cellular products such as digestive enzymes to muscular activity, which, via peristalsis, propels a meal along the tube of the alimentary tract. Carbohydrates constitute the medium-term energy fuel, often taken by athletes as 'carbohydrate loading' before an event. Long-distance muscle fuels are provided by fatty acids and triglycerides, which enable the skeletal muscles to maintain activity over a protracted length of time. Therefore, if we ingest energy fuels, such as carbohydrates and fats, and they are not used for physical work, either metabolism or physical activity, they will be deposited in the fat stores within the adipocytes (which see below).

DISORDERS OF EATING

The need to eat a balanced diet

We also eat to enable growth and repair: in addition to the energy fuels, a balanced diet must include protein, which is needed for cellular regeneration and repair. Proteins are chains of amino acids. Some amino acids can be synthesised by the liver but others have to be included in the diet to avoid deficiency, hence their description as **essential amino acids**.

Other components of a balanced diet include **water**, the medium for chemical reactions, transport and maintenance of normal body temperature, and inorganic elements, including **electrolytes** such as sodium, potassium and calcium, which are used among other purposes for nerve conduction and muscle contraction. **Vitamins** are chemicals that are used in a range of reactions: some act as coenzymes in the chemical cascade reaction during which ATP is produced. Vitamins are either water-soluble (vitamins B and C), or fat-soluble (vitamins A, D, E and K). Figure 4.1 indicates some of the range of activities of the vitamins.

Fibre is another component of a normal diet. Although it cannot be used for metabolic processes, it is needed to stimulate peristalsis within the alimentary tract and its presence influences the absorption of certain other dietary substances such as iron.

As humans are omnivorous creatures, the dietary requisites can be

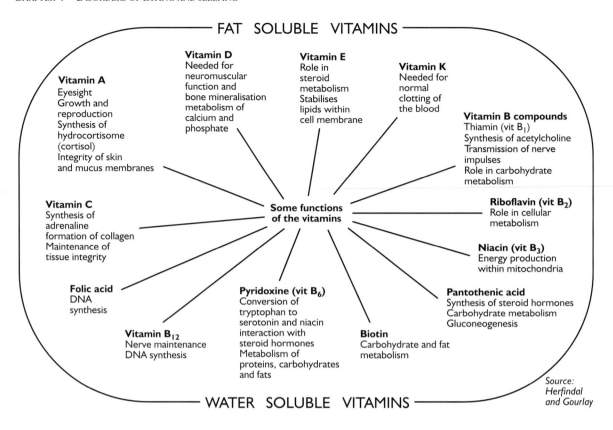

Figure 4.1

Some of the roles of vitamins

obtained fairly easily as long as a varied food intake is maintained. Unfortunately, foods containing a high proportion of fats are appealing to many in the Western world: if these endurance fuels are not used for the purpose for which the body was designed to use them (physical work), then excessive accumulations of fat stores ensues. Obesity is a form of malnutrition and is a particular problem, both in adults and children, in the so-called developed countries.

Key point ▶

> In order to maintain a normal body composition, the amount of energy taken in as the diet must be equal to the amount of energy expended on metabolic or physical work.

Glucose

Glucose is a particularly important nutrient as it forms the major energy source of the cells of the nervous system. Whatever the nutritional state of the body at any given time, the brain must receive its energy substrate. Accordingly, when food is not being taken into the body, for example during the night, a steady release of glucose from the glycogen stores of the liver occurs under control of the hormone glucagon, and this stored glucose is used for cerebral metabolism. When the glucose supplies are low, one feels the cerebral effects of this, a sense of shakiness, anxiety and hunger. (See also the section on Diabetes mellitus in Chapter 8.)

This period without intake of food is termed the **fasting phase** of metabolism, and at such times the brain is literally being kept alive by the activity of the liver in releasing stored glucose from the glycogen store.

Once we awake and eat more food, the metabolic processes enter the **absorptive phase**. Among other nutrients, glucose suddenly becomes in abundant supply, and it is possible to allow its uptake by all body cells. As the blood glucose levels rise, insulin is produced by the beta cells of the islets of Langerhans in the pancreas. Insulin enables glucose to be taken up by all body cells for use as energy. Unfortunately, as well as relishing dietary fats, people enjoy the taste of simple carbohydrates – if there is more glucose in the blood than is needed for the creation of cellular energy, then the glucose will join the fatty acids and glycerol in the adipocytes as the liver converts the excess into energy stores.

An interesting phenomenon is seen when a sugary 'snack' is taken. The manufacturers' advertising material usually advocates the benefits of such foodstuffs for allaying hunger between meals. Unfortunately, the opposite process tends to occur: the snack is eaten and the blood glucose levels rise. This causes secretion of insulin into the bloodstream, which enables the sugar to enter the cells and the blood glucose level drops correspondingly. This produces an overshoot effect: as the glucose level decreases, the sense of hunger returns as strongly as ever, causing the person to wish for (and possibly, eat) another sugary treat. This is good news for the snack manufacturers, but less so for the eater, who may soon require a new size in clothes due to the burgeoning fat stores!

Prolonged fasting

Should food not be taken at the appointed time, the hepatic stores of glucose are largely consumed and other measures are needed to keep the brain and body alive. Activity levels can be decreased so less intake is needed. Dieters may discover, to their frustration, that, if they reduce their diet to a marked degree, they become lethargic and it becomes more of an effort to expend energy. They also begin to use the fat stores in the adipose tissues. Fatty acids and glycerol are released from the stores in the adipocytes. The glycerol is converted by the liver into glucose for cerebral metabolism and the fatty acids are used by the remaining body cells. If prolonged fasting occurs, the state of **starvation** is imminent and the body must seek alternative fuels. As a last resort, protein can be used to provide cellular energy, and tissues such as muscle are broken down to this end. When the constituent amino acids of a protein chain are broken down for energy, keto-acids are produced, which can be detected in the urine. This starvation state produces muscle wastage, so now the person appears emaciated as there is no adipose tissue and muscle mass is being used as maintenance fuel.

Readers who work with clients with anorexia nervosa (see below) will be familiar with this picture.

Key point ▶

> In health, energy use is carefully balanced against the availability of energy fuels. Different phases of metabolism exist that maintain energy homeostasis when food is scarce or in abundant supply.

What makes us eat?

It is thought that one in four people in western Europe is obese (Carter, 1998). Because of the incidence of obesity in Western society, much scientific activity is being directed to trying to understand what it is that controls appetite, and what happens when we are hungry. Certainly, most of us are habituated to expect to eat at certain times, and this is fuelled by social and environmental factors. People who are used to living with another person who is no longer there may lose the drive to eat, and the pain of loss may be made worse by the reminder that only half the amount of food needs to be prepared and only one place at the table is needed. This encourages the omission of the whole distressing ritual of food preparation and consumption. It is interesting for most people in the Western world to consider when they last ate a meal simply because they were hungry. Other reasons for eating may include the fact that the meal 'was there' or because another person expected the food they had prepared to be eaten. Sometimes, out of politeness (or self-preservation), such food is eaten with appropriate signals of gratitude and enjoyment even if the meal itself is quite unpalatable!

Key point ▶

> Many behavioural and social influences govern the drive to eat.

The generation of hunger

There is an array of cues that stimulate the sensation of hunger. There are the environmental factors previously described, such as time of day. There are factors related to the sensory system, such as the sight, sound or, most importantly, the smell of food being prepared. The sight of an appealing type of food may generate a drive to eat because the food was 'fancied', even though physical hunger was not present at that time. People will eat more if variety is offered, as, interestingly, will laboratory rats! People will also eat more if they need to make only a minimal effort to get the food; hence convenience foods and snacks and delicious meals cooked by someone else are probably the main culprits in causing the current epidemic of obesity in the affluent areas of the world.

The drive to eat was obviously one of the earliest behaviours developed during evolution. Within the brain two areas, the area postrema and the nucleus of the solitary tract, receive information from the tongue, stomach and intestines and from the liver and the brain

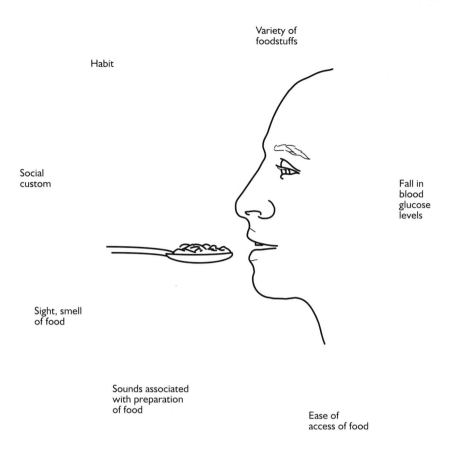

Habit

Variety of
foodstuffs

Social
custom

Fall in
blood
glucose
levels

Sight, smell
of food

Sounds associated
with preparation
of food

Ease of
access of food

Figure 4.2

Factors increasing the drive to eat

itself in relation to glucose levels. The information received is forwarded to the forebrain, where specific areas control eating. Information from the tongue and organs of the alimentary tract is also passed to the pons, although the role of the brain stem in this context is not well known. Figure 4.2 summarises factors influencing hunger.

Protection against starvation

The lateral hypothalamus contains neurones that influence eating. One group of neurones increases hunger and reduces the metabolic rate, thus conserving stored nutrients. Research with mice has revealed that these neurones secrete the peptide neurotransmitters melanin-concentrating hormone (MCH) and orexin. The presence of either MCH or orexin in the lateral ventricles of the brain is associated with increased eating; a deficiency is associated with suppression of food intake. Axons of the nerves that secrete these two transmitters have been found to synapse with a range of cerebral structures that influence motivation and movement.

When there is a shortage of glucose or lipids, the MCH- and orexin-secreting neurones are stimulated by neurones that secrete neuropeptide Y, another transmitter. When administered experimentally to rats, neuropeptide Y stimulates avid feeding. When present in the lateral hypothalamus, neuropeptide Y promotes eating. When present in the medial hypothalamus, in the paraventricular nucleus that surrounds part of the third ventricle, neuropeptide Y produces a series of responses related to conserving nutrients: insulin and cortisol are secreted, release of fats from adipocytes is inhibited and body temperature is reduced. Neuropeptide Y seems to be associated with stimulating eating: food deprivation increases the levels of this transmitter and eating reduces its concentration. The axons of neuropeptide Y fibres innervate areas of the brain influencing metabolism as well as synapsing with orexin and MCH neurones that influence eating.

Box 4.1

The anti-starvation transmitters: summary of the functions of neuropeptide Y, orexin and melanin-concentrating hormone

- Neuropeptide Y
  - Stimulates eating
  - Inhibits metabolic function and thus energy use in times of nutritional deprivation
  - Suppresses gonadotrophin thus inhibiting ovulation and sexual responsiveness
  - Contributes to control of insulin secretion
  - Decreases metabolic rate
- Melanin-concentrating hormone (MCH) and orexin
  - Increase food intake
  - Decrease metabolic rate

As indicated above, hunger is mediated within the hypothalamus, where the lateral and ventromedial nuclei have the ability to generate or suppress the drive to eat. Incoming signals from the sensory system interact with the area of the hypothalamus that generates the hunger response.

A sequence of hormones prepares each part of the alimentary tract in turn for the arrival of a meal. The salivary glands moisten the mouth to ensure adequate lubrication and the presence of salivary amylase for the initial work on digestion of cooked starch. It is no coincidence that appealing food is described as 'mouth-watering'! Further hormones prepare the stomach for the arrival of food, hence the rumbling from increased peristalsis that may occur in consequence. Following on in sequence, under the influence of gut–brain transmitters and hormones such as cholecystokinin, the duodenum, gall bladder and segments of the small intestine are sequentially activated to receive the chyme, which is the result of homogenised food mixed with digestive juices. Finally, some hours later, the colon extracts water and electrolytes and the rectum is activated to void the residue as faeces.

Experimental attention has been paid to the possible influence of fluctuations of levels of specific nutrients in the blood. It appears that eating is modulated by various categories of signal that provide information about short- and long-term nutritional status. The blood levels of particular nutrients such as glucose are monitored by receptors in the brain and liver. Thus, levels on each side of the blood–brain barrier are monitored, by the liver on the outside and by the brain on the inside. If blood sugar levels fall, hunger is experienced. The long-term reservoir of 'endurance fuels' (fat and fatty acids) is within the cells of the adipose tissue. Although it easy to think of adipose tissue as an inert tissue rather like the lagging round a boiler, in fact adipose tissue possesses mechanisms enabling communication with systems that control eating and nutrient levels in the blood (Figure 4.4).

As can be seen from Figure 4.4, there is a nerve supply to the tissue. Sympathetic nerve fibres stimulate the adipocytes to release fatty acids and glycerol if there appears to be a need for rapid mobilisation and escape from danger. Even though most of the modern-day threats are not successfully avoided by this strategy, the old fright or flight mechanisms still work. There is also a blood supply to adipose tissue, into which hormones can be secreted from the adipocytes to inform the control centres of the current status of the long-term fuel store. Severe depletion of the lipid store produces hunger, but this hunger is most marked when both glucose and lipids are in short supply. It may be that receptors for glucose and lipids exist within the cells themselves. This reasoning is based upon the fact that, in poorly controlled diabetes mellitus, the blood glucose levels are abnormally high while the patient feels very hungry: some signalling mechanism must be indicating that the cells are starving in the midst of energy fuel that cannot be accessed because of inability to transport the glucose across the cell membrane. It is also possible that changes in cellular metabolic rate influence the development of sensations of hunger.

There is also experimental evidence (Carlson, 2001) to suggest that a system of monitoring the levels of specific nutrients via intestinal nutrient detectors may exist. Work with rats deprived of specific foodstuffs resulted in the rats being observed to seek out and eat preferentially foods consisting of the missing nutrients.

◀ **Key point**

> A whole system of structures exist to monitor short- and long-term nutritional status, within the brain, within the circulation and, probably, within the cells.

What makes us stop eating?

The sense of having eaten sufficient to reduce any further drive to eat is called satiety. Lack of readiness of the alimentary tract to receive food has an inhibitory effect upon the sense of hunger. Older people tend to secrete less saliva and less digestive juices, which has an influence upon the drive to eat: if the mouth feels dry and food seems to become 'stuck' as chewing takes place, then it is easy to see why food, particularly that presented in comparatively large amounts, can become a disincentive to eat. Stretch receptors are present in the stomach and other areas of the alimentary tract: the feeling of being full up is usually a potent inhibitor of the drive to eat any more. If the lack of adequate peristalsis causes the stomach to empty slowly, resulting in a feeling of being bloated, then this again produces a disincentive to eat. Information related to the level of nutrition prior to eating a meal will determine whether a lot or a little will be eaten before satiety is experienced. If a person or an animal has not eaten for a long time, then they will eat for longer before the hunger is appeased.

Satiety is controlled by a range of factors, which are introduced below.

Head factors

These factors involve information from receptors in the nose (smell), tongue (taste), throat and eyes. Sensations related to the sight, smell, taste and texture of food contribute towards satiety, particularly for specific categories of food. At the cinema, someone might have had enough salted popcorn but quite fancy an ice cream, although these foodstuffs in themselves will not of course contain the ingredients of a balanced diet!

Gastric factors

Although stretch receptors within the stomach exist, hunger and satiety are experienced even if the stomach has been surgically removed. Therefore information from the stomach can only contribute to the sense of satiety. Experimental work has demonstrated that animals can regulate the food they choose to eat according to its calorific value and their present energy needs (Carlson, 2001). Within the stomach and intestines, specific nutrient receptors have been identified that control ingestion of particular nutrients within the diet.

Intestinal factors

Axons that respond to concentrations of amino acids, fatty acids and glucose have been found in the duodenum. These are thought to contribute to the feelings of satiety for specific nutrients. It has also been found that the duodenum secretes cholecystokinin, a hormone that regulates the rate at which the stomach empties as well as stimulating the gall bladder to expel bile into the common bile duct and thus into the duodenum. Cholecystokinin is secreted in response to the presence of fats in the duodenum. Injected cholecystokinin has been found to produce a temporary suppression of eating and is also thought to take effect via cholecystokinin receptors, which are concentrated on the pylorus, thus acting at the junction between the stomach and the duodenum. A good explanation of current experimental work related to the control of hunger and satiety is to be found in Carlson, 2001.

The role of the liver

The liver receives proof that food has been absorbed as plasma nutrient levels rise. Experimental work has indicated that the liver has receptors for glucose and fructose. When levels of these nutrients are elevated in

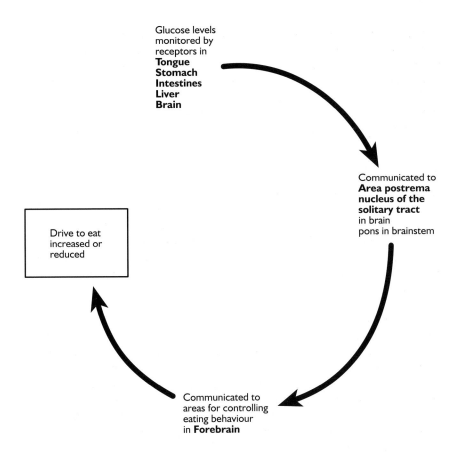

Glucose levels monitored by receptors in
Tongue
Stomach
Intestines
Liver
Brain

Communicated to
Area postrema
nucleus of the
solitary tract
in brain
pons in brainstem

Communicated to areas for controlling eating behaviour in **Forebrain**

Drive to eat increased or reduced

the hepatic capillaries, it appears that information confirming satiety is sent to the areas of the brain that control appetite. The role of receptors in many areas associated with eating is shown in Figure 4.3 in relation to control of glucose levels.

> Specific nutrient receptors within parts of the alimentary tract send feedback to the brain about the exact nutritional status within the body.

◄ **Key point**

Long-term monitoring of nutritional status

Communication about nutrition has so far related to the consumption of specific meals. In addition, the brain gathers intelligence about long-term trends in nutrition, particularly in relation to total body fat content. The question of how the brain normally knows how much fuel is held within the fat store is of obvious interest in relation to helping people with obesity. Work with a strain of mice that are naturally obese has enable researchers to identify leptin, a hormone which is secreted into the bloodstream when adipocytes have quantities of stored triglycerides (Figure 4.4).

Figure 4.4

The mechanism by which adipose
tissue communicates with the brain

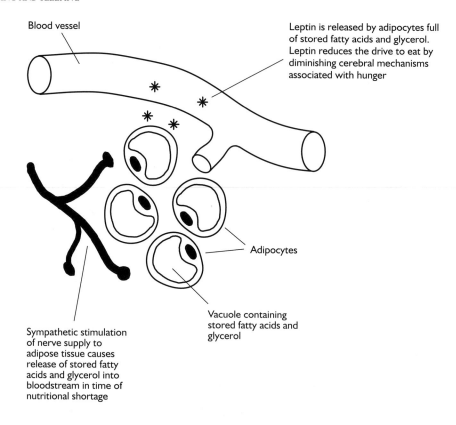

Blood vessel

Leptin is released by adipocytes full
of stored fatty acids and glycerol.
Leptin reduces the drive to eat by
diminishing cerebral mechanisms
associated with hunger

Adipocytes

Vacuole containing
stored fatty acids and
glycerol

Sympathetic stimulation
of nerve supply to
adipose tissue causes
release of stored fatty
acids and glycerol into
bloodstream in time of
nutritional shortage

As may be been seen in Figure 4.4, when the adipocytes are filled
with stored triglycerides, the cells secrete the hormone leptin into the
bloodstream. This hormone is thought to sensitise the hypothalamus to
signals of satiety and thus inhibit further eating. It may be that people
who are markedly obese have reduced sensitivity to leptin: the brain
simply fails to respond to signals that food intake can for the present be
reduced as there are considerable energy stores laid by in the adipose
tissue.

Key point ▶

> Adipose tissue secretes leptin, a hormone which indicates that fat
> stores are high and that eating can be reduced.

The ventromedial hypothalamus has an important role in the control
of body composition, mobilising nutrients during fasting. It communi-

Key point ▶

> When little food is being taken, the ventromedial hypothalamus acts
> via the vagus nerve to reduce parasympathetic activity, decrease
> insulin production and increase secretion of glucagon, adrenaline
> (epinephrine) and noradrenaline (norepinephrine). This reduces the
> activity of the alimentary tract and stimulates the release of glucose
> and fatty acids from store.

cates with areas of the brain, such as the nucleus of the solitary tract, that receive information about nutrient levels from the tongue, alimentary tract and liver. It also communicates with the parts of the vagus nerve that regulate insulin secretion.

The role of the central nervous system in satiety

As discussed above, the hormone leptin is released by adipocytes that are replete with stored fats. The result of leptin binding with receptors in the brain is to inhibit eating and to increase the metabolic rate. Leptin receptors are also present on neurones that secrete neuropeptide Y (the peptide that greatly stimulates eating). When leptin binds to these neurones, their rate of firing is inhibited, so eating is suppressed. The opposite effect occurs when glutamate, another transmitter substance, binds to neuropeptide-Y-secreting neurones. In such instances, the presence of glutamate stimulates the normal response to fasting – increased hunger and reduced metabolic rate.

Leptin mediates the response to the well-fed state: eating is decreased and the metabolic rate in increased. Glutamate mediates the response to fasting: eating is increased, metabolic rate is diminished.

◀ *Key point*

Another neuropeptide has been found to inhibit eating. In the mid-1990s, a peptide was discovered that increases when cocaine or amphetamines (amfetamines)are taken. For this reason, the peptide was called cocaine- and amphetamine-regulated transcript (CART). Levels of CART in the brain fall in conditions of food deprivation and rise in times of sufficiency. CART neurones suppress eating and increase the metabolic rate, so, like leptin, they mediate eating in times of high food availability. CART neurones also contain leptin receptors, so the two transmitter systems are apparently interlinked.

Leptin inhibits neuropeptide Y neurones, suppressing eating and increasing metabolic rate. Leptin also stimulates the activity of CART, which in turn causes the suppression of MCH and orexin neurones which would otherwise produce an appetite increase. It is thought that CART receptors in the spinal cord may help to produce the rise in metabolic rate caused by leptin. The role of leptin is related to long-term appetite suppression as a result of dietary excess. Cholecystokinin works in conjunction with leptin to inhibit eating. Serotonin also has an appetite-suppressant effect and serotonin-secreting neurones are thought to work in conjunction with the cholecystokinin mechanism. Drugs that inhibit the action of serotonin increase eating, especially of carbohydrates.

The three disorders discussed below, obesity, bulimia nervosa and anorexia nervosa, all involve loss of normal control of food intake. Although it is not classed as a mental health disorder, an overview of obesity is considered first. A useful review of eating disorders is available in Thompson (2001) and Dawson (2001).

Obesity

As explained above, a range of mechanisms normally exist that control eating in relation to the amount of food available and the extent of stored fat within the adipose tissue. Body composition can be assessed by dividing the weight in kilograms by the square of the height in metres to arrive at the **body mass index**. A normal body mass index is between 19 and 25. Less than 19 is underweight, between 26 and 30 is overweight and more than 30 constitutes obesity.

It is apparent simply by looking around that the Western world is facing a considerable increase in the incidence of obesity. At its most basic level, to maintain a normal body fat content, the amount of food taken in must be balanced against the levels of energy expended. As has also been explained, numerous complex neural mechanisms exist to control eating appropriately for the prevailing nutritional state. Nowadays, concern about safety has meant that children tend to be driven to school, rather than arriving under their own steam. When they get home, they may have a convenient snack consisting of sugary or fatty foods. Then, instead of engaging in play involving gross motor activity, they may turn to computer-generated games that involve only sedentary activity. Their parents also may exercise little and eat a diet heavily skewed to fats and sugars. Thus, energy intake outstrips energy output and the fat stores in adipose tissue increase. Long-term obesity is associated with insulin resistance, and this has now been found to be developing in teenagers, rather than the older adult as was previously the case. Although genetic and psychosocial factors are likely to play a part in the current epidemic of obesity, it appears as if some neuro-chemical failure may also be to blame.

Key point ▶

> Current-day lifestyles, particularly for children, tend to involve insufficient energy output to balance the dietary input. The incidence of obesity is increasing.

Various treatments for obesity exist, the most simple and obvious being to decrease the energy intake of food and increase the energy output in the form of exercise. A range of surgical techniques exist that are designed to reduce the efficiency of the alimentary tract in digesting and absorbing nutrients. These are outside the scope of this book. Dietary measures in which non-absorbable fats are substituted for dietary fats are used by some to control obesity, and these have the attraction that many of the products are commercially available, so the sufferer can access them directly. Unfortunately, some of these have the unpleasant side-effects of causing flatulence and diarrhoea. A proportion of dietary fat is needed to build new phospholipid molecules for cell membranes. Cholesterol is also needed for construction of cell membranes and for synthesis of steroid hormones, so a balanced nutritional state will not be achieved by banning fats of all sorts from the diet.

New knowledge of how appetite and satiety are mediated has not yet been fully applied to enhance understanding of obesity, but offers promising future approaches to management.

Drugs used in the treatment of obesity

There is much competition among pharmaceutical companies to create effective appetite-suppressing substances. In the past, amphetamines have been used for this purpose: these agents raise the metabolic rate and suppress appetite but they are addictive and so pose their own health hazards. Serotonin suppresses appetite and serotonin agonists are sometimes used as part of a weight-control strategy. **Fenfluramine** is an example of a serotonin agonist that has been used to control appetite, although its use has decreased because of the potentially hazardous side-effects of lethargy, depersonalisation, pulmonary hypertension and depression on withdrawal of the treatment. **Dextrofenfluramine** and **fluoxetine** now tend to be used instead.

It is likely that the results of research on the neural mechanisms governing the stimulation and suppression of appetite may lead to a breakthrough in the treatment of obesity. Until then, most treatments have the problem that they do not help the client to alter his/her eating patterns or activity levels. Supportive psychological therapy or group sessions, conducted by organisations such as Weight Watchers, are aimed at helping the client to gain better lifestyle control as part of a healthier approach to living.

Eating disorders requiring specific mental health care

People with eating disorders have been categorised in relation to their personality types (Westen and Harnden-Fischer, 2001). From this exercise, three subgroups were identified: high-achieving perfectionists; people who appeared constricted and overcontrolled; and a third group who were emotionally dysfunctional and undercontrolled. Westen and Harnden-Fischer recommend that the personality pathologies should be taken into account as well as the nature of the eating disorder, as both anorectics and bulimics may have a variety of personality dysfunction and an incomplete profile is possible if a client is categorised simply according to the psychiatric diagnosis.

> Personality traits need to be taken into account as well as the medical diagnosis of eating disorders.

◀ *Key point*

Bulimia nervosa

Bulimia is predominantly a condition affecting young females in Western countries. The physical appearance of a person with bulimia nervosa tends to be relatively unremarkable. There is a characteristic fluctuating pattern of binge eating and then the use of purging or vomiting to remove the ingested foodstuffs from the body. Binge eating is defined as the consumption of more food than would be ingested by normal people in similar circumstances over a similar amount of time.

Bulimics tend to identify certain foods as being 'forbidden' or 'junk foods' and these are chosen for episodes of immoderate eating. In preparation, the bulimic person may go out to buy a large supply of the foods. Often, quite a sum of money is spent in the process. Once the food is brought home, it may be thrown away so as to avoid eating it. Food bought for a binge-eating spree tends to contain items, such as yogurt or ice cream, that are easy to swallow and vomit. During an eating binge extreme amounts of food, involving proteins and fats as well as carbohydrates are ingested.

People with early bulimia tend to eat their food extremely rapidly; as the condition becomes well established the food is eaten more slowly as long as the risk of being discovered is considered to be comparatively slight. In these cases, very small amounts of food may be taken over a protracted period of time. Thousands of calories may be eaten in this way. Added to the urge to overeat, vomiting or purging through the use of laxatives is employed to avoid the fat deposition that would normally accompany such a massive energy intake. Accompanying this collection of behaviours is a fear of becoming overweight.

Bingeing–purging behaviour can also be a characteristic of a form of anorexia nervosa (see below).

It is relevant here to differentiate the effects of bulimia nervosa from those of binge-eating disorder, in which the use of vomiting or purging is not present. Both conditions are associated with a loss of control. Binge-eaters may use exercise or dieting to maintain control over body weight. Table 4.1 differentiates the characteristics of bulimia nervosa and binge-eating disorder.

It is thought that those who use purging as a means of weight control have a greater disturbance of their body image and an increased level of anxiety related to eating. It is considered that around half of people with bulimia self-induce vomiting, either by putting their fingers down their throats to produce gagging or by voluntarily producing a contraction of the abdominal muscles and diaphragm. Such people may suffer electrolyte or nutritional imbalances and repeated vomiting is associated with erosion of tooth enamel and damage to the oesophagus due to acid reflux.

The incidence of bulimia is greater than that of anorexia and it is becoming more common. It is thought that the true number of those suffering from some form of bulimia is underestimated because of a disinclination to present for treatment or to disclose the existence of their problem.

A range of factors is associated with the development of a bulimic episode. Anxiety, boredom, use of alcohol, going out with a member of the opposite sex and coming home from school or work are associated with an eating binge. Some degree of psychological instability is often

Bulimia nervosa	Binge-eating disorder
Recurrent binge eating	Recurrent binge eating
Sense of loss of control over eating	Sense of lack of control over eating during the binge
Excessive amount of food eaten within a given time period	
Inappropriate behaviour to retain control over body composition, for example induced vomiting or purging	At least three of the following present: • Eating more rapidly than usual • Eating until distension causes discomfort • Large amounts eaten in the absence of hunger • Lack of planned meal times • Embarrassment and avoidance of eating with others because of quantity of food eaten • Depression, disgust or guilt related to the binge
At least two episodes of binge eating and two examples of inappropriate weight-control activities each week over a minimum period of 3 months	Generally binge-eating occurs at least twice a week over any 6-month period
Preoccupation with body weight and shape	Distress caused by the condition
May or may not be associated with anorexia nervosa	No use of laxatives or dieting medication

Table 4.1

Differences between bulimia nervosa and binge-eating disorder (adapted from Szmukler et al., 1995).

present, demonstrated by labile mood, impulsiveness, anxiety and reduced tolerance of frustration. A loss of self-esteem is commonly present. Bulimics seem to have a tendency to be part of disorganised or otherwise dysfunctional families who have high expectations of achievement. There may be a sense of loss of control, which is compensated by dieting and weight loss. Bulimia may first present after an episode of dieting or loss of or separation from a significant person.

The effect of food cues upon bulimic subjects has been examined by Neudeck et al. (2001), who found that, irrespective of the blood sugar level at the time, subjects who were presented with high-calorie food experienced greater stress and a stronger urge to binge-eat than did subjects who were presented experimentally with low-calorie food.

> A bulimic eating binge involves consumption of abnormally large amounts of food over a given time span. This may occur through gorging or through constant ingestion of very small amounts of high calorie food. Vomiting or purging may or not be part of the pattern.

◀ *Key point*

As is to be expected, the role of neurotransmitters related to eating has been the subject of scrutiny by researchers. The effects of dieting upon plasma levels of the serotonin precursor L-tryptophan and levels of serotonin within the brain have been examined by Cowen and Smith (1999). These researchers' findings in women indicate that dieting is associated with a reduction in L-tryptophan, the onset of depressive symptoms and increased concern about weight, body shape and fear of loss of control of eating. Cowen and Smith suggest that, in susceptible people, these changes are sufficient to trigger the onset of bulimia nervosa.

Bulimia is associated with reduced serotonin metabolites in cerebrospinal fluid and suggestions have been made that it is associated with decreased serotonin use in the brain, that endocrine responses are associated with downregulation of postsynaptic serotonin receptors and that hypersensitivity to serotonin receptors that control gastric sensations may exist. As considered earlier, serotonin is known to inhibit behaviour associated with eating and serotonin activity is reduced when chronic dieting is undertaken. An interesting study into the effects of serotonin upon some of the symptoms associated with bulimia nervosa was undertaken by Steiger *et al.* (2001), who concluded that bulimia is associated with a generalised disorder of serotonin regulation. It is also thought that there is a change in levels of noradrenaline (norepinephrine) in the brain in this illness.

Treatment of bulimia

In a double-blind, placebo-controlled trial, Hudson *et al.* (1998) found that, despite the associated adverse reactions of this preparation, **fluvoxamine** was associated with a reduction in the frequency of eating binges in sufferers from binge-eating disorder. Other workers (Mitchell *et al.*, 2001) evaluated **fluoxetine** and found that the use of this selective serotonin reuptake inhibitor (SSRI) in conjunction with a self-help manual was effective in reducing vomiting and the incidence of binge-eating episodes in adult women with bulimia nervosa. In an Austrian study evaluating **reboxetine**, an antidepressant with a selective noradrenaline reuptake inhibitor action, over a period of 12 weeks, this agent was found to reduce the incidence of binge eating and vomiting episodes (El-Giamal *et al.*, 2000). **Inositol**, another agent normally used to treat depression, panic disorders and obsessive–compulsive disorder (OCD), has been suggested to be of potential value in the treatment of bulimia nervosa and binge-eating (Gelber *et al.*, 2001).

Hence, a range of agents are being tried to help treat the client with bulimia. A Cochrane Review of the respective merits of antidepressants versus placebo in the treatment of bulimia nervosa by Bacaltchuk and Hay (2002) suggests that, in general, antidepressants can make an effective contribution to the treatment of clients with bulimia nervosa, that no one class of antidepressant is really outstanding, but that fluoxetine presents an acceptable treatment in many cases.

As with obesity, the increased understanding of the neurophysiology of appetite control is likely to lead to new directions in the treatment of this group of conditions, although, as with many mental health disorders, the cause is probably multifactorial and pharmacological treatment will need to be part of a wider strategy that includes social and psychological approaches. The problem of loss of personal control indicates that clients need help to regain their ability to self-determine and this is unlikely to be achieved solely by pharmacological means.

CASE STUDY 4.1	JANICE – A NICE EVENING AT HOME

Read this case study and then attempt to answer the questions that follow.

Janice has just got home from the shops. Laden with carrier bags, she enters the house she shares with friends. Everyone else is out for the evening. Janice unloads her purchases: four litre tubs of vanilla ice cream, two moderate-sized gateaux, a family-sized bar of chocolate and a large pack of potato crisps. She lays out a series of small spoons and a knife, she'll just try out the food she has bought, so she collects it all on to a tray, goes into the sitting room and switches on the television.

Three hours later, Janice looks at the time – 11pm. She also looks around her – empty wrappers and cartons everywhere! She finds a black rubbish bag, puts all the litter into it and takes the bag out to the dustbin. Hmm, she has rather overdone it! She finds her laxative tablets: better take a triple dose. By the time her flat mates come in, Janice is in bed. Yes, she's fine, she has enjoyed her evening. No, she didn't go out, unfortunately, she has another of her 'stomach upsets' .

1. What factors might have predisposed to Janice's bulimia?
2. Is the misuse of laxatives of any particular significance?
3. In a person with normal control of their eating, what mechanisms would be likely to have curtailed Janice's eating spree?
4. Does Janice need help?

Anorexia nervosa

This condition is characterised by extreme fear of fatness and weight gain. The anorectic is often a young female, although the incidence of anorexia nervosa in males is increasing. The pursuit of thinness is undertaken in disregard of the evidence of emaciation in the mirror before the sufferer, and comes to dominate all aspects of that person's life. The theme of control plays a significant role in the activities of the anorectic person, whose goals are geared towards dieting to attain ever lower body weights. To this end, dieting may be augmented by slimming preparations, purgatives or vigorous exercise.

Because in the female the development of the secondary sexual characteristics and menstruation are closely associated with gaining a threshold level of adipose tissue within the body composition, theories have been offered that anorexia nervosa is closely bound with avoidance of mature female sexuality. However, these ideas are contentious, and anorexia nervosa does affect males as well as females, although less commonly. Although some authorities at one time considered that bulimia nervosa was a stage of deterioration in anorexia nervosa, it is now thought that the two conditions are separate, although related to a certain extent, particularly in anorectics who exhibit a habit of bingeing and purging or inducing vomiting. Some authorities divide anorectics into those who maintain control by restricting their diet and those who eat excessively and then purge themselves or induce vomiting to avoid weight gain. In the established anorexia sufferer, considerable subterfuge may take place as the person wears loose clothing to conceal the extent of their thinness. During weighing sessions the impression of weight gain may be given by previously drinking large quantities of water or by concealing weights upon the person.

Key point ▶

> Anorexia nervosa occurs in males as well as females.

Since the 1960s, there has a been a culture in which thinness in women has been prized. A range of role models and toys such as 'Barbie' dolls have helped to instil the notion that thinness is desirable. An interesting study in Finland (Rintala and Mustajoki, 1992) examined the shape of shop-window models and found that, since the 1960s, the types of body composition represented by the models would, if they had been alive, have comprised insufficient adipose tissue to support ovulation. In other words, they were presenting an ideal of a sterile female.

Anorexia nervosa is comparatively common in ballet schools, where thinness is prized as part of the 'ideal dancer' shape. These ideas were demonstrated in the 1990s by the director of a British national ballet company who complained that British dancers were the wrong (pear) shape to look elegant in performance. There is little wonder then that young female dancers may resort to heavy cigarette smoking to maintain their weight (smoking increases the blood sugar and therefore suppresses hunger) and, in addition, take to using excessive weight control measures.

People with anorexia nervosa are not necessarily repelled by food: considerable interest in the preparation of food may exist, particularly if a meal is being prepared for others. It seems to be the prospect of weight gain after eating that is the concern of the anorexic person. Links have been made between anorexia nervosa and obsessive–compulsive disorder. Depression and sleep disturbance may be present.

Key point ▶

> The incidence of anorexia nervosa is probably fuelled by the prevailing culture in which thinness is valued.

Various theories exist regarding the physiological causes of anorexia nervosa. One school of thought implicates a disorder of hypothalamic neurotransmitters and failure of neuroendocrine regulation. Others have suggested that these neurochemical alterations result from the state of starvation that results. There is much written discussion of the psycho-social causation of anorexia nervosa, but this is a specialist subject in itself and beyond the scope of this book. Some experts suggest that heredity plays a significant part in the causation of the condition.

Studies of changes in neurotransmitters suggest that noradrenaline, serotonin and endogenous opioid levels become abnormal in anorexic people. Researchers have identified elevated levels of neuropeptide Y (see above) in the cerebrospinal fluid of people with severe anorexia. This may account for the weight loss, preoccupation with food and cessation of menstruation in severely underweight sufferers.

Anorexic people who are seriously underweight have diminished levels of leptin in their cerebrospinal fluid. There seems to be an abnormality of the leptin system. Normally, it will be recalled, leptin signals to reduce appetite when the adipose tissue is well stocked with stored fats. It is surprising, therefore, that in anorexia nervosa, the leptin levels normalise long before the proportion of body fat returns to anywhere near normal amounts. As a result, appetite is suppressed early in the refeeding programme, which makes it difficult for the anorexic patient to comply with nutritional goals. Theories also exist that, in anorexia, dopamine activity within the hypothalamus may be excessive.

◀ **Key point**

> In anorexia the disordered body image is compounded by dysfunction of the normal neurochemical signalling mechanisms which are part of nutritional homeostasis.

Pharmacological treatment of anorexia nervosa
Many preparations have been tried as treatment for anorexia nervosa but few have been entirely successful. At best, they are adjuncts to psychological therapies aimed at shaping the behaviour towards normal eating and restoring the weight to a level that will sustain life. In cases where the client is in a state of starvation, the first priority of care is to prevent death and to improve the nutritional status. Measures to try to reorganise the anorectic person's attitudes and values regarding his/her body image necessitate the use of therapeutic strategies. For appropriate discussion of these, the reader is referred to a text such as Thompson, 2001.

As will be seen below, a range of pharmacological agents have been tried but care of anorexic clients is doomed to failure unless permanent attitude adjustment can be achieved. Long-term anorexia is associated with a series of health risks due to the persistent state of starvation. Apart from infertility, a range of problems such as hepatic damage, osteoporosis and increased susceptibility to infection may reduce the client's quality and length of life.

Medication has been used in an attempt to relieve symptoms of anorexia nervosa, to correct supposed biochemical imbalances and to induce compliance with treatment. In addition, drugs have been used in an attempt to produce a direct weight gain (although these last strategies raise issues of ethical acceptability). One suspects in such cases that, once the medication was discontinued, unless significant attitude change had occurred, the client would take pains to lose the weight again.

When drugs are indicated, great care is needed with the dosage and care should be taken to watch for signs of toxicity. This is because the starvation state may produce renal or hepatic impairment and the abnormal body composition may alter drug distribution within the body. Should liver impairment cause a reduction in plasma proteins, carriage of protein-bound drugs may also be less predictable. Because of the specific problems of body weight in these clients, precise drug dosages will not be generally stated in this section.

Key point ▶

> The poor nutritional condition in severe anorexia nervosa means that much drug therapy is hazardous and so is not undertaken lightly.

Anorectic clients who are receiving treatment to try to restore normal nutritional intake are sometimes handicapped by feelings of abdominal distension. The reason for this is that gastric emptying tends to be slower, causing food to tend to accumulate in the stomach and produce the counterproductive sense of being bloated. **Metoclopramide** is an antiemetic agent that increases the rate of gastric peristalsis, so it hastens gastric emptying and relieves clients of the unpleasant and, for them, particularly distressing symptom of gastric distension. Metoclopramide also is thought to antagonise dopamine in the hypothalamus, which also raises the possibility that its use would help to correct some of the biochemical abnormalities of this condition.

Metoclopramide may cause extrapyramidal symptoms, particularly if used in conjunction with neuroleptic medication. Spasm of the facial muscles, with tongue protrusion and speech disturbances, and overall increase in muscle tone may occur. In overdose, metoclopramide may cause disturbance of muscle tone.

A proportion of clients with anorexia nervosa also have symptoms of depression. This may be because aspects of anorexia may in themselves produce depression; because anorexia nervosa involves disturbance of the same neurotransmitter systems that produce depression; or because the state of starvation produces a mental state similar to depression. There seems to be a lack of studies evaluating the use of antidepressants in anorexia nervosa, although fluoxetine has been suggested to be useful in helping the client to maintain his/her target weight once eating has been successfully re-established (Szmukler *et al.*, 1995). **Amitriptyline** has been used by some for anorexic clients as this agent induces a craving for carbohydrates and produces weight gain, although, again, the ethics of this treatment may give cause for concern.

Amitriptyline can produce adverse reactions, which malnourished patients are more likely to suffer. If a malnourished person is to receive tricyclic antidepressants, they need prior screening for cardiovascular, renal and hepatic function, and usually receive a low initial dose, which is then gradually increased.

Anorectic people often have issues related to personal power and control, so may not be willing to take prescribed medication. For further information relating to antidepressant agents, see Chapter 3.

> Treatment of anorexia nervosa is geared around nutritional rehabilitation and supportive therapy to maximise the effectiveness of this.

Other medication used in the treatment of anorexia nervosa
Dopamine blockers have been tried in response to the theory of dopamine excess as a cause of this condition. However, the results do not at present indicate demonstrable therapeutic benefits. Because anxiety is a common feature of anorexia nervosa, neuroleptic agents have been used. In early days, **chlorpromazine** was used in association with insulin. People with anorexia nervosa have increased sensitivity to insulin, and hypoglycaemia has the effect of causing hunger. In nutritionally compromised people, the dose of chlorpromazine should not exceed 300 mg daily and should be given for short periods only. Insulin treatment is not currently favoured because of the hazards associated with induced hypoglycaemia (hypoglycaemic coma and death). **Thioridazine** has also been used (Szmukler *et al.*, 1995) Weight gain was achieved but, as has been discussed, the treatment has hazardous side-effects. Probably, good nursing care would be as effective in achieving a safer improvement in nutritional status.

Minor tranquillisers such as **lorazepam** 0.25–0.5 mg are sometimes given about an hour before meals to reduce anxiety in anticipation of eating. This can be useful when the client is in the early stages of reinstitution of eating, or if s/he is facing a specific situation that is known to cause worry or to exacerbate the anorexia. For further information on benzodiazepine tranquillisers, see Chapter 2.

Cyproheptadine, a serotonin and histamine antagonist, has been used in the hope of reducing the metabolic rate and stimulating weight gain, although there remains a lack of positive evidence of its benefit. Endogenous opioids such as endorphin (naturally occurring painkilling molecules) have been suggested as having a role in appetite regulation. Use of **naloxone**, the antagonist to opioid analgesia, has been tried but not been seen to exert any beneficial effect upon the appetite. Given in association with amitriptyline and anticonvulsants, some have found this to be effective but it is expensive and must be administered as an intravenous infusion, making its use less acceptable to the client and posing hazards related to infection. Similarly, lithium, which is known to increase body weight and regulate mood, has been tried, but it appeared that there was little therapeutic benefit to justify the risk of using such a potentially toxic preparation for such a physiologically vulnerable client group. Anticonvulsant agents such as **phenytoin** and **carbamazepine** have also been tried, to induce weight gain in anorectics who binge eat. Further detail related to anticonvulsant agents may be found in Chapter 8.

Zinc sulphate has been used with some success to improve weight and appetite. The basis of this treatment is that zinc lack is associated with nausea and aversion to food. Unfortunately, zinc salts can cause dyspepsia and abdominal pain which could prove counterproductive when trying to encourage anorectic subjects to eat. In overdose, zinc causes irritation and ulceration of the mucosa of the mouth and stomach, so induction of vomiting is contraindicated should a client take excessive amounts of this preparation.

As with bulimia nervosa, as knowledge increases of the biochemical factors inherent in anorexia nervosa, pharmaceutical treatment of this condition may gain greater prominence. However, the complexity of the condition is such that skilled therapeutic support is likely to remain centrally important in the treatment of this potentially lethal illness which at present remains difficult to treat.

CASE STUDY 4.2   **JACQUETTA, A CLIENT WITH ANOREXIA NERVOSA**

Read this case study and then attempt to answer the questions that follow.

Jacquetta is a 16-year-old student. She has just left school and is now studying window display at the local Further Education college. She had hoped to be an international-level gymnast but didn't quite make the grade, which disappointed her father who used to coach her. She likes college and her new friends; collectively, they have a reputation among the other students for being cool trend-setters. The current fashions suit Jacquetta, although she does wish she wasn't so fat. She usually wears black, with a baggy overshirt to conceal the extra inches, which she suspects are the real reason why she failed to make it into the international squad. If only she could lose another 5 kilograms! Jacquetta considers herself something of an expert on food and she controls her calorie intake meticulously. Of course she eats. At meal times, her plate is piled high with carrot sticks, raw cauliflower and lettuce and tomato slices, which she takes a long time to eat as she chews it all very methodically, 25 times for each mouthful. It's sometimes hard to eat all of her meal, as she feels rather full by the time she is half way through. Twice a day, Jacquetta works out. Early in the morning she jogs before her breakfast of two apples. When she gets back from college, she goes to the gym, where she does high-impact aerobics. People make such a stupid fuss about her – her mother has this fixation that she is too thin and must visit the doctor, when really, she is *so huge!*

1. What factors need to be taken into account when considering Jacquetta's case?
2. Is Jacquetta's mother likely to be acting unreasonably?
3. Who could help and what could they do?

SLEEP

Although sleep has been intensively studied, its exact nature and functions remain incompletely understood. Sleep is a universal experience. We know instinctively that we need a certain amount of sleep, also that if we sleep too much or too little we do not feel at our best. This need to have adequate sleep may at times become an overwhelming preoccupation.

Key point ▶ | Sleep remains an incompletely understood phenomenon but inappropriate quantities of sleep are generally thought to be associated with impaired performance.

Sleeping and waking

Various areas of the brain and neurotransmitters are involved with maintaining a normal pattern of sleeping. In order for sleep to commence, arousal must be reduced. The pons and the reticular activating system are involved with sleep induction, as are the neurotransmitters serotonin and acetylcholine. The cycles of sleeping and waking are usually synchronised within a circadian rhythm associated with levels of light. The hormone melatonin, released by the pineal gland when light levels are low, is associated with reduced activity levels and sensations of sleepiness.

> Sleep appears to occur as a result of interaction between environmental circumstances, neurones in specific parts of the central nervous system and selected neurotransmitters.

◀ **Key point**

Control of the phases of sleep

The mechanisms by which the phases of sleep are controlled are not completely understood. As benzodiazepine drugs, which bind to gamma-aminobutyric acid (GABA)$_A$ receptors, produce sleepiness, it is likely that a naturally occurring molecule that binds to these same receptors has a role in the control of sleep. However, such a substance has yet to be discovered. Production of adenosine within the ventro-lateral preoptic area of the brain (part of the forebrain close to the hypothalamus) has also been suggested to have a role in the production of drowsiness, sleep and the delta wave activity in slow-wave sleep (SWS). If injected experimentally into the basal forebrain, adenosine has been observed to increase the time spent sleeping. Sleep induction also appears to be linked in some way to brain temperature. Neurones within the ventrolateral preoptic area are thought to secrete GABA and thus to inhibit areas of the brain such as the tubomamillary nucleus, raphe nuclei and locus ceruleus, all areas that, when activated, cause cortical arousal and active behaviour (Carlson, 2001).

Rapid-eye-movement (REM) sleep is controlled by structures within the pons. REM sleep is inhibited during SWS by neurones secreting serotonin within the raphe nuclei and by noradrenaline (norepinephrine)-secreting neurones within the locus ceruleus. Acetylcholine levels in the cerebral cortex have been found to be at their highest levels during waking and REM periods and at their lowest levels during SWS. REM sleep is initiated in the dorsolateral pons by acetylcholine-secreting neurones. A state of muscular paralysis is produced that seems to prevent the sleeper from acting out dreams. At the appropriate point in the sleep cycle, REM sleep is inhibited by neurones that secrete noradrenaline and serotonin.

Stages of sleep

It is thought that the timing of the phases in the sleep cycle is controlled within the medulla oblongata. A normal period of sleep consists of a series of different types of physiological activity, each accompanied by characteristic electrical activity as observed on an electroencephalogram.

In Stage 1 sleep, there is the sense of losing concentration and control of eye movements and, if the individual is sitting upright, perhaps in a situation when alertness is needed, there is an embarrassing loss of control of neck and jaw muscle tone. If the sleeper is being observed in a sleep laboratory, characteristic changes in the electroencephalogram (EEG) appear: the EEG waveform becomes larger and slower as the sleep cycle progresses from stage 1 to stage 2 sleep and from that to stage 3 and stage 4 sleep. The cycle of sleep varies in length between species: the larger the brain the longer an individual sleep cycle lasts. In rats the sleep cycle is around 12 minutes; in humans the cycle lasts 90 minutes and is repeated a number of times during the overall period of sleeping. Figure 4.5 shows the cycle of sleep.

Stage 4 SWS (also called non-rapid-eye-movement or NREM sleep) is characterised by a large, slow EEG waveform. The person appears 'dead

Figure 4.5

The sleep cycle

(a)   EEG when awake

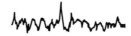

(b)   Cycle of sleep

Stage 1   Dropped off relaxed: vague thoughts, drowsiness, very easily awoken.

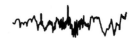

Stage 2   More relaxed. Vague dream-like thoughts. Obviously asleep, but easily awoken.

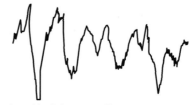

Spindle

Slow wave or non-REM sleep

Stage 3   Complete relaxation. Slowing of pulse and other bodily functions. Not woken by background noise.

Stage 4   Complete relaxation, little movement. Difficult to awaken.

REM sleep. Deep sleep. Vivid dreaming. Characteristic eye movement.

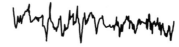

to the world', moves little and undergoes slowing of vital functions such as heart and respiratory rate. During SWS, increased levels of human growth hormone are released into the bloodstream and there are changes in the levels of the immune stimulant interleukin-1, which appears to induce sleep in addition to increasing the white cell count. This observation has fuelled the suggestion that SWS has a role related to maintenance of normal immunity and that it is also needed for tissue growth and repair. The individual is deeply asleep and it seems that, during this phase, the cerebral cortex is temporarily isolated from somatic stimuli.

Slow-wave sleep is influenced by structures within the nucleus of the solitary tract and the circuit between the thalamus and the cerebral cortex (Keshavan *et al.*, 1998). Interestingly, when a baby is rocked to soothe it , this activity is thought to stimulate the same area of the brain (Carlson, 2001).

The amount of time spent in SWS drops markedly from the third decade of life. SWS seems to occur less in people who suffer sensory deprivation and it has been noted that less SWS also occurs people who suffer from clinical depression and that some people with schizophrenia have no noticeable episodes of the characteristic SWS delta waveforms. SWS deprivation studies have shown little apparent effect apart from the subject developing a slightly greater tendency to focus upon minor bodily symptoms and to have an increased tendency to feel depressed.

To the casual observer, perhaps the most obvious stage of sleep is REM sleep. This phase of the sleep cycle is controlled in the pons. The effects of REM sleep can be easily observed – twitching of the limbs and jaw and eye movements are obvious as the skeletal muscle depolarises. Staff on night duty may have to suffer the effects of some patients in REM sleep grinding their teeth. Although REM sleep is 'deep', the sleeper can be roused if called by name and, on waking, is fully alert. (Carlson 2001).

The exact function of REM sleep is not entirely clear, although it is during this phase that dreaming occurs. Interesting theories relating to the function of REM sleep include the suggestion that it is needed for some sort of mental organisation of recent experiences so as to form memories and to establish or modify learned behaviour patterns (Kunz and Hermann, 2000). The same authors suggest that sleep has a role related to energy storage within the brain. It has also been suggested that, during REM sleep, repairs previously made to the neuronal structure are tested and that any redundant neural connections are removed to increase cognitive capacity. It has been observed that REM sleep occurs in greater amounts following a period of intensive learning. Strength is given to these theories by the absence of this type of sleep in more primitive species.

Experimental deprivation of REM sleep appears to produce little noticeable effect apart from a slight tendency to social withdrawal and feelings of suspicion and insecurity (Horne 1988).

Key point ▶

Although there seem to be no dramatic results if the sleep patterns are interrupted, it appears that subjects report such sleep to be in some way of lesser quality in comparison to normal sleep.

As the period of sleeping progresses, the time spent within the various stages changes, with the majority of the SWS occurring during the early part of the sleep period and increasing amounts of REM occurring in the later stages of the sleeping time. Figure 4.6 is a schematic representation of the architecture of a night's sleep. During the process of awakening, the noradrenergic neurones increase their rate of firing, which contributes to the return of the state of normal wakefulness.

Box 4.2

Dreaming

- Dreams occurring in rapid-eye-movement sleep tend to be experienced in the form of 'stories'
- Dreaming can also occur in slow-wave sleep, but tends rather to produce experiences, such as the sensation of being crushed.

Figure 4.6

Architecture of a night's sleep

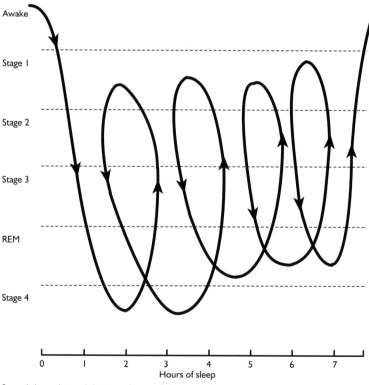

Stage 4 sleep obtained during early part of sleep period
4-6 sleep cycles completed during sleep period
Progressively more time spent in REM as night progresses.

SLEEP DISORDERS

A wide range of sleep disorders exist and any may have adverse effects upon the quality of life of the sufferer. Within this section, sleep disorders that are associated with mental health problems will be considered, the wider subject of altered sleep being beyond the scope of this book.

Insomnia

Virtually every adult has experienced difficulty with sleeping at some stage in their life. Individual needs for sleep very greatly, so insomnia is best individually defined as a significant decrease in the amount or quality of sleep compared to what is normal for that person. The sleep of a person suffering from insomnia may not be qualitatively different from that of a 'normal' sleeper but it is perceived as inadequate. Insomnia may take the form of difficulty in falling asleep (delayed sleep onset), repeated awakenings from sleep, or early wakening, with the sufferer waking several hours before usual and then being unable to return to sleep. Insomnia may be acute or chronic, associated with taking or withdrawal from a particular form of medication, substance dependence, or with being troubled by mental, social or physical problems. Sleep disturbance may be associated with depression, schizophrenia or bipolar disease.

Some sufferers who lose the 24-hour circadian pattern of sleep may be helped by light therapy (Watanabe *et al.*, 2000). Sufferers from insomnia are well advised to try non-pharmacological ways of achieving sleep but, if these are ineffective, they may be prescribed hypnotic agents – drugs that induce sleep. Although the client's experience is then of restored sleep, the quality of the sleep differs from the normal sleep architecture so the natural pattern of delta slow-wave and REM sleep may be lost when treatment with hypnotics is prescribed. This can cause rebound reactions and a paradoxical deterioration in sleep, which may be a particular problem for elderly clients requiring pharmacological assistance to restore sleep. Phototherapy (treatment with bright light) may be of benefit to patients with certain forms of insomnia (Hori *et al.*, 2000).

The pattern of sleeping and waking occurs in roughly 24-hour cycles and during this time the sleeper passes through different levels of sleep that recur in cycles. There is a suggestion (Gruber *et al.*, 2000) that children with attention-deficit hyperactivity disorder have an imbalance in their sleep–wake system. Major depression may be associated with a breakdown in the integral rhythms that characterise a normal period of sleep (Armitage *et al.*, 1999). Shift work has been identified as disrupting the normal circadian timing of sleeping and waking, and this in turn has been associated with the development of clinical depression in some vulnerable individuals (Scott, 2000). It is possible that some sections of the population have particular difficulty in compensating for sleep loss, which disrupts their circadian rhythm and results in delayed sleep phase syndrome (Uchiyama *et al.*, 2000).

Key point ▶

> Sleep disturbance may be associated with a variety of mental illnesses.

Some members of the population suffer from **hypersomnia** (excessive sleepiness), which may be due to a failure of the normal arousal mechanisms and which may be successfully treated with CNS stimulants (Vgontzas *et al.*, 2000).

Hypnotic agents

In order to induce sleep, it is necessary to use a substance that suppresses CNS activity. Any delayed excretion will result in residues of such agents being present in the brain during the daytime and will produce psychomotor slowing and drowsiness during waking. For these reasons, clients newly using hypnotics may need advice about avoiding situations such as driving or using other hazardous machinery when their vigilance is reduced.

Benzodiazepines

These agents are commonly used to induce sleep. Problems were found with some agents, as REM suppression plus rebound sleep disturbances such as insomnia occurred on cessation of treatment (for further detail, see the section discussing benzodiazepines for treatment of anxiety in Chapter 2).

Flurazepam 15–30 mg induces sleep and is slowly metabolised without causing rebound problems due to the suppression and subsequent rebound of REM sleep. However, flurazepam interferes with delta SWS and this tends to result in daytime drowsiness, particularly in older people.

Temazepam in doses of 15–30 mg helps to increase the total sleep time and to reduce sleep fragmentation. Both temazepam and **triazolam** tend to reduce REM sleep in the first half of the sleep period but then to compensate during the later stages, which reduces perceived sleep disturbance. Triazolam seems not to interfere with delta sleep, so reduces the morning 'hangover' effect and daytime drowsiness, and has an overall beneficial effect upon the perceived quality of sleep.

Other hypnotic agents

Benzodiazepine receptor agonists

Zolpidem is a hypnotic agent that acts by binding to benzodiazepine-1 (BZD_1) receptors. In a daily dose of 10 mg (5 mg for elderly clients), it is used in the short-term treatment of insomnia. Because of its specific affinity for BZD_1 receptors, it produces a strong hypnotic effect but lacks the muscle relaxant, anxiolytic amnesiac and anticonvulsant effects of benzodiazepines and does not affect delta sleep. Zolpidem reduces sleep latency (time taken to fall asleep) increases sleep time and reduces sleep fragmentation (awakenings during the period of sleep). It is less susceptible to abuse than the benzodiazepines and does not produce rebound insomnia when the client ceases treatment. It is not suitable for clients with psychotic illness because, as with benzodiazepines, zolpidem may cause restlessness, agitation, irritability, inappropriate behaviour or hallucinations or other psychotic reactions. Overdosage causes drowsiness or light coma.

Future developments

Pharmacologically induced sleep tends to differ from natural sleep because of interference with the normal sleep phases. The ideal hypnotic agent would restore both normal length and quality of sleep.

Application of the science of chronobiology (the effect of time upon biological systems) may yield further helpful aids to sleep restoration. Investigators in the Netherlands and Japan (Nagtegaal *et al.*, 2000; Kamei *et al.*, 2000) have independently evaluated the use of the hormone **melatonin** as having potential value as treatment for sufferers from sleep-phase syndrome. A new generation of sleep-inducing agents based upon hormones and other sleep-inducing natural molecules may in future offer a more natural form of therapeutically-induced sleep.

Somnambulance

Somnambulance (sleepwalking) occurs in slow-wave (delta) sleep. It particularly affects young children, who usually grow out of the condition. Its relevance to this text is that sleepwalking may be provoked by medication such as lithium, fluphenazine and desipramine. Drugs such as benzodiazepines that suppress delta sleep have the potential to reduce sleepwalking in adults who have frequent hazardous sleepwalking episodes.

Sleep terrors

Sleep terrors affect a small number of children and an even smaller number of adults. The sleeper wakes in a state of extreme disturbance, screaming, with rapid pulse and respiratory rates, and has a sense of intense fear, but no recall of the content of the dream. Children usually outgrow the condition; adults for whom this condition is a problem could in theory be helped by suppression of delta sleep by the use of benzodiazepines.

Nightmares

Nightmares occur in a percentage of the population (around 5%) who wake recalling a complex, frightening dream. Rebound nightmares occur in people who are withdrawing from drugs that suppress REM sleep as part of their mode of action. Suffers from post-traumatic stress disorder suffer from nightmares that may in future be usefully treated with **cyproheptadine**, a serotonin-2 antagonist that has properties similar to antihistamine. However, the use of this agent remains contentious at present (Rijnders *et al.*, 2000; Jacobs-Rebhun *et al.*, 2000).

Narcolepsy

This is a relatively rare condition in which the sufferer experiences extreme daytime sleepiness. Hypnogogic hallucinations (a bizarre dream-like state in the transition between sleep and waking) may occur, and cataplexy and sleep paralysis (muscular weakness that may cause the sufferer to collapse before sleep occurs) may be distressing features of this condition. Narcolepsy is thought to be a disorder of REM sleep: sufferers make a transition directly between full wakefulness and REM sleep without passing through the interim stages. The paralysis results from the muscular effects of REM sleep. Episodes of narcolepsy may be triggered by emotional stimuli such as anger, laughter or excitement.

It appears that there is a genetic basis to the condition. Workers in California (Bourgin *et al.*, 2000), have identified excitatory neuropeptides called hypocretins that act within the locus ceruleus and are involved in the development of REM sleep and the pathophysiology of narcolepsy. This knowledge may lead to a new pharmacological treatment for this condition. CNS stimulants such as antidepressants and, recently in the USA, modafinil have been used to treat this condition.

Box 4.3 Sleep apnoea	The symptoms of this condition are caused by interrupted sleep resulting from airways obstruction by the tongue or other anatomical abnormality of the throat. Obstruction of the airflow produces a characteristic pattern of snoring, which reaches a crescendo; breathing may then cease for a period of time until carbon dioxide accumulation and oxygen lack produces partial awakening and resumption of the breathing pattern. Depending upon the nature of the sleep apnoea, the individual may complain of daytime sleepiness, or insomnia, as of course may their unfortunate partner!

SUMMARY

The concept of balance occurs repeatedly in this book. In this chapter we have considered the natural balancing mechanisms that control eating and sleeping. A range of mechanisms govern the activity of eating and the maintenance of adequate energy stores. Eating disorders are increasing in incidence and frequently involve issues related to control and anxiety, the individual's personality and the prevailing social culture and customs. Advances in the understanding of neurochemical signalling mechanisms are helping mental health professionals to develop ways of helping people with obesity or bulimia; anorexia nervosa at present is more responsive to psychological than to pharmacological treatment. Although sleep is a universally experienced phenomenon, its exact nature remains obscure. Sleep disorders accompany many mental illnesses; pharmacological treatment restores sleep to some extent but the quality differs from that of natural sleep.

REFERENCES AND FURTHER READING

Armitage, R., Hoffmann, R.F. and Rush, A.J. (1999) Biological rhythm disturbance in depression: temporal coherence of ultradian sleep EEG rhythms *Psychological Medicine*, **29**, 1435–1438.

Bacaltchuk, J. and Hay, P. (2002) Antidepressants versus placebo for people with bulimia nervosa (Cochrane Review). In: *The Cochrane Library*, issue 1. Update Software, Oxford.

Bourgin, P., Huitron-Resendiz, S., Spier, A.D. *et al.* (2000) Hypocretin-1 modulates rapid eye movement sleep through activation of locus ceruleus neurons. *Journal of Neuroscience*, **20**, 7760–7765.

Carlson, N.R. (2001) *Physiology of Behaviour*, 7th edn. Allyn & Bacon, Boston, MA.

Carter, R. (1998) *Mapping the Mind*. Phoenix, London.

Cowen, P.J. and Smith, K.A. (1999) Serotonin, dieting, and bulimia nervosa *Advances in Experimental Medicine and Biology*, **467**, 101–104.

Dawson, D. (2001) *Anorexia and Bulimia: A Parents' Guide to Recognising Eating Disorders and Taking Control*. Vermilion, London.

El-Giamal, N., de Zwaan, M., Bailer, U. *et al.* (2000) Reboxetine in the treatment of bulimia nervosa: a report of seven cases. *International Clinical Psychopharmacology*, **15**, 351–356.

Gelber, D., Levine, J. and Belmaker, R.H. (2001) Effect of inositol on bulimia nervosa and binge eating. *International Journal of Eating Disorders*, **29**, 345–348.

Gruber, R., Sadeh, A. and Raviv, A. (2000) Instability of sleep patterns in children with attention-deficit hyperactivity disorder. *Journal of the American Academy of Child and Adolescent Psychiatry*, **39**, 495–501.

Hori, T., Watanabe, T., Kajimura, N. *et al.* (2000) Effects of phototherapy on the phase relationship between sleep and body temperature rhythm in a delayed sleep phase syndrome case. *Psychiatry and Clinical Neurosciences*, **54**, 371–373.

Horne, J. (1988) *Why We Sleep: The Functions of Sleep in Humans and Other Mammals*. Oxford University Press, Oxford.

Hudson, J.L. McElroy, S.L., Raymond, N.C. *et al.* (1998) Fluvoxamine in the treatment of binge-eating disorder: a multicenter placebo-controlled, double blind trial. *American Journal of Psychiatry*, **155**, 1756–1762.

Jacobs-Rebhun, S., Schnurr, P.P., Friedman, M.J. *et al.* (2000) Posttraumatic stress disorder and sleep difficulty. *American Journal of Psychiatry*, **157**, 1525–1526.

Kamei, Y., Hayakawa, T., Urata, J. *et al.* (2000) Melatonin treatment for circadian rhythm sleep disorders. *Psychiatry and Clinical Neurosciences*, **54**, 381–382.

Keshavan, M.S., Reynolds, C.F. III, Miewald, M.J. *et al.* (1998) Delayed sleep deficits in schizophrenia: evidence from automated analysis of sleep data. *Archives of General Psychiatry*, **55**, 443–448.

Kunz, D. and Hermann, W.M. (2000) Sleep-wake cycle: sleep-related disturbances and sleep disorders: a chronobiological approach. *Comprehensive Psychiatry*, **41**(Suppl 1), 104–115.

Mitchell, J.E., Fletcher, J., Hanson, K. *et al.* (2001) The relative efficacy of fluoxetine and manual-based self-help in the treatment of outpatients with bulimia nervosa. *Journal of Clinical Psychopharmacology*, **21**, 298–304.

Nagtegaal, J.E., Laurant, M.W., Kerkhof, G.A. *et al.* (2000) Effects of melatonin on the quality of life in patients with delayed sleep phase syndrome. *Journal of Psychosomatic Research*, **48**, 45–50.

Neudeck, P., Florin, I. and Tuschen-Caffier, B. (2001) Food exposure in patients with bulimia nervosa. *Psychotherapy and Psychosomatics*, **70**, 193–200.

Rijnders, R., Laman, D.M. and van Diujn, H. (2000) Cyproheptadine for posttraumatic nightmares. *American Journal of Psychiatry*, **157**, 1523–1525.

Rintala, M. and Mustajoki, P. (1992) Could mannequins menstruate? *British Medical Journal*, **305**, 19–26.

Scott, A.J. (2000) Shift work and health. *Primary Care: Clinics in Office Practice*, **27**, 1957–1979.

Stahl, S.M. (1996) *Essential Psychopharmacology: Neuroscientific Basis and Practical Applications.* Cambridge University Press, Cambridge.

Steiger, H., Young, S.N., Kin, N.M.K. *et al.* (2001) Implications of impulsive and affective symptoms for serotonin function in bulimia nervosa. *Psychological Medicine*, **31**, 85–95.

Szmukler, G., Dare, C. and Treasure, J. (1995) *Handbook of eating disorders. Theory, treatment, and research.* John Wiley & Sons, Chichester.

Thompson, J.K. (2001) *Body Image, Eating Disorders and Obesity in Youth: Assessment, Prevention and Treatment.* American Psychological Association, Washington, DC.

Uchiyama, M., Okawa, M., Shibui, K. *et al.* (2000) Poor compensatory function for sleep loss as a pathogenic factor in patients with delayed sleep phase syndrome. *Sleep*, **23**, 553–558.

Vgontzas, A.N., Bixler, E.O., Kales, A. *et al.* (2000) Differences in nocturnal and daytime sleep between primary and psychiatric hypersomnia: diagnostic and treatment implications *Psychosomatic Medicine*, **62**, 220–226.

Watanabe, T., Kajimura, N., Kata, M. *et al.* (2000) Case of a non-24h sleep-wake syndrome patient improved by phototherapy. *Psychiatry and Clinical Neurosciences*, **54**, 369–370.

Westen, D. and Harnden-Fischer, J. (2001) Personality profiles in eating disorders: rethinking the distinction between Axis I and Axis II. *American Journal of Psychiatry*, **156**, 547–562.

Websites

Anorexia nervosa: http://www.netdoctor.co.uk/diseases/facts anorexianervosa.htm
Bulimia nervosa: http://www.mentalhealth.com/icd/p22-et02.html
Insomnia: http://www.pslgroup.com/INSOMNIA.HTM
Sleep apnoea: http://www.britishsnoring.demon.co.uk
Narcolepsy: http://www.uic.edu/depts/cur/

SELF-TEST QUESTIONS

Identify the correct statements in the following questions. For each question, some, all or no options may be correct.

1. You wake up late and go to work without breakfast. Which of the following statements are true?
    a. you will be secreting insulin so as to move more glucose into the cells
    b. your liver must release glucose from glycogen stores
    c. you are likely to lose weight
    d. the adrenaline (epinephrine) produced in the process of rushing to work is the fuel that keeps you going
2. Which of the following factors contribute to a feeling of satiety (being 'full up')?

    a.   activation of stretch receptors in the stomach

    b.   increased gastric peristalsis

    c.   lack of variety in type of foods eaten

    d.   secretion of cholecystokinin.

3.   Which of the following statements are true in relation to obesity?

    a.   there is a familial influence

    b.   fluoxetine has appetite-suppressant properties, making it of use in the treatment of obesity

    c.   raising the metabolic rate will increase obesity

    d.   lifestyle control is an important part of treatment

4.   Which of the following statements about bulimia nervosa are true?

    a.   if a bulimic client buys 'junk food' she always eats it

    b.   bulimic people tend to put a lot of effort into food preparation

    c.   an eating binge commonly involves only one kind of foodstuff

    d.   a fear of becoming overweight is often the basis of bulimia nervosa

5.   A client has bulimia nervosa. Which of the following statements about the condition are correct?

    a.   bulimia nervosa is a more commonly occurring condition then anorexia nervosa

    b.   in this condition, increased serotonin usage occurs within the brain

    c.   depression in bulimia nervosa may be associated with reductions in the levels of L-tryptophan

    d.   bulimic sufferers are commonly the subjects of high family expectations

6.   Which of the following statements apply to Jennifer, who is a seriously underweight client with anorexia nervosa?

    a.   she may engage in obsessive preparation of food

    b.   she may be noticeably hyperactive

    c.   she may experience feeling of being bloated due to delayed gastric emptying

    d.   she is likely to consider herself to be overweight

7.   Jennifer's plan of treatment is likely to include:

    a.   a physical health assessment

    b.   use of tricyclic antidepressants

    c.   medication to slow peristalsis

    d.   strategies to increase her nutritional intake

8.   Which of the following are involved with the phases of normal sleep?

    a.   cerebral temperature

    b.   decreased secretion of melatonin

    c.   production of adenosine

    d.   secretion of gamma-aminobutyric acid

9.   Which of the following mental health problems commonly accompany sleep disorders?

    a.   bipolar affective disorder

    b.   depression

     c.   general anxiety disorder

     d.   schizophrenia

10. Which of the following statements are correct?

     a.   somnambulance (sleepwalking) can occur if a client takes lithium

     b.   substance dependence can be associated with insomnia

     c.   hypnotic substances restore the normal sleep architecture

     d.   hypersomnia can be successfully treated with CNS stimulants

SCHIZOPHRENIA

5

INTRODUCTION

The characteristics of schizophrenia were first collectively described about 100 years ago by a German psychiatrist, Emil Kraepelin. He noticed a group of patients who shared a variety of symptoms and a tendency to deteriorate over time and coined the term 'dementia praecox'. Eugen Bleuler, in 1908, criticised the term dementia praecox, stating that there was no global dementing process. He first used the term 'schizophrenia' and formed the basis of the diagnostic criteria that are in use today.

Schizophrenia is characterised by disturbances of thinking and perception and is often associated with shallow or inappropriate emotions. Insight, the ability of an individual to recognise that they have a mental illness, may also be lacking.

The costs of schizophrenia to patients, their families and society are overwhelming. Patients can suffer from life-long debilitating symptoms; families often carry the burden of care; and society has to meet the substantial direct and indirect costs of the illness. The aetiology of schizophrenia remains elusive, in part because it is likely that many factors are responsible for the manifestation of symptoms. An underlying genetic predisposition to the illness may be triggered by factors such as viral infections and birth complications. One hypothesis postulates that an insult to the brain that occurs early in neurodevelopment produces symptoms of the illness at a later point in the individual's development.

Despite a lack of understanding of the pathophysiology of schizophrenia, the 1950s saw a major breakthrough in the treatment of the illness with the introduction of a drug called chlorpromazine. This drug was the first to actually bring relief by reducing the effects of hallucinations and delusions. It heralded the beginning of a move towards treating people with schizophrenia in the community. Many new drugs have followed that are not only more effective but also lack many of the distressing side-effects associated with the earlier drugs. These will be discussed in further detail later in the chapter. Advancing technology will greatly increase our understanding of schizophrenia in the years to come, with the likelihood of better treatments and improved quality of life for our patients. There are already claims that the newer, so-called atypical antipsychotics will reduce the clinical deterioration associated with this neurodegenerative disorder.

CLINICAL PICTURE

Schizophrenia is a relatively common mental disorder, having a lifetime prevalence of around 1%. Annually, 7500 patients are newly diagnosed with schizophrenia in the UK and they cost UK society an estimated £862 million in the 5 years following diagnosis (Guest and Cookson 1999). Costs attributable to the National Health Service account for 38% of the total. For many, schizophrenia is a disabling mental illness that is characterised by impairment of insight and contact with reality and in which there is great heterogeneity in the symptoms, course and outcomes. This diversity is not only seen in different individuals but also in the same individual over time. Schizophrenia is not about having a split personality, nor does bad parenting or personal weakness cause it. It is a disease, or more probably, a collection of diseases, with a physical cause.

Key point ▶

> Approximately 1% of the population will develop schizophrenia during their lifetime.

Schizophrenia often follows a chronic relapsing course, although about a quarter of people with the disorder experience a remission after a single or just a few psychotic episodes (Lieberman 1996). Many will become chronically ill, with frequent relapses disrupting periods of relative normality, while others will be symptomatic for much of the time and are referred to as having 'treatment-resistant' schizophrenia.

Onset can be either insidious or acute. Before the illness can be diagnosed there is often a period of increased tension and poor concentration. Sleep may be affected and the person can find maintaining friendships, work and even personal care increasingly difficult. Many individuals drop out of work or education, producing high unemployment among this group. Certain features of schizophrenia such as clumsiness and movement disorders may even be noticeable in childhood long before the symptoms necessary for diagnosis become evident.

The course of schizophrenia can be divided into phases (Figure 5.1). The first phase is the **premorbid phase** – in other words, the phase characterised by a lack of any evidence of the illness. That is not to say that the premorbid phase is non-pathological. Neurodevelopmental changes may be occurring in response to environmental influences long before the first signs of the illness become apparent. Attempts to identify antecedents to later morbidity may help target at-risk individuals for early health promotion activities.

Key point ▶

> The course of schizophrenia can be divided into four phases, the premorbid phase, the prodromal phase, the active phase and the residual phase.

The premorbid phase is followed by the **prodromal phase**, which generally occurs during adolescence. During this time there may be early warnings of impending illness characterised by subtle, non-specific

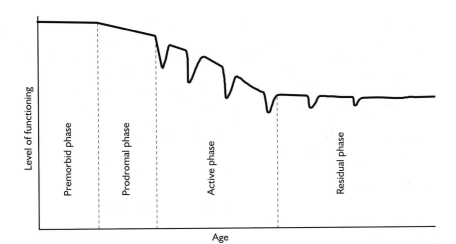

Figure 5.1

Phases of schizophrenia

symptoms. While these symptoms, such as low mood, irritability and social withdrawal, are not confined solely to schizophrenia, their presence is thought to be related to the later emergence of the illness. The importance attached to the identification of prodromal symptoms lies in the need for early intervention, now widely recognised as significant for improved outcome.

The prodromal phase precedes the **active phase**, the formal onset of the illness where a diagnosis is made. The active phase tends to be the most chaotic. The majority of patients recover from their first psychotic episode, although further episodes often lead to a progressive deterioration in functioning. This phase can last many years before the symptoms become dominated by the cognitive and negative symptoms of the **residual phase**. By this phase, further psychotic episodes are unlikely to produce significant further decline in functioning.

The prognosis for individuals diagnosed with schizophrenia is impossible to predict with any certainty. However, a lack of premorbid symptoms; abrupt onset, typically during middle age; a predominance of florid symptoms and a lack of blunted affect; and early medical and social intervention are associated with a better long-term prognosis.

Both sexes are affected equally by the illness, although the age of onset tends to be slightly earlier in men, generally between the ages of 18 and 25 years, as opposed to 25–30 years for women. Schizophrenia can also develop later in life and it has been known in children as young as 9 years of age. Some studies suggest that women experience a less severe and different pathological process of schizophrenia and propose that oestrogens may confer protection (Castle *et al.*, 1995). Other research has found gender differences in the size of the temporal lobe in patients with schizophrenia. Magnetic resonance imaging (MRI) comparisons found that men with schizophrenia had a significantly smaller temporal lobe than men without schizophrenia, whereas similar comparisons with women showed little difference in temporal lobe size

(Sheringham, 1999). This may shed light on why men and women respond differently to medication and have different clinical profiles in schizophrenia (Sheringham, 1999). Some 10% of people with schizophrenia will eventually commit suicide (Caldwell and Gottesman 1992).

Key point ▶

> Gender differences in schizophrenia include age of onset and severity of symptoms. Women often experience their first symptoms later than men, and these symptoms may be less severe.

Schizophrenia is a psychotic disorder: in other words, symptoms of psychosis are its defining features. Psychosis itself is not a disorder but a syndrome, which includes the symptoms of delusions, hallucinations and disorganised speech and behaviour. Other disorders, including depression and Alzheimer's disease, may involve symptoms of psychosis but these are not required for diagnosis.

Schizophrenia is characterised by distortions of thinking and perception, and by inappropriate or blunted affect. Consciousness and intellectual capacity are generally unaffected by the illness, although in time cognitive deficits may become apparent. Affected individuals may experience intrusion of their thoughts and feelings, believe that they are at the centre of everything that happens, and develop bizarre delusional ideas that provide explanations for their odd behaviour. Hallucinations are common, although perception can be altered in other ways: the importance attached to colours, sounds and objects can be disproportionate to their actual significance. Those affected can also become perplexed, believing that everyday situations have great meaning to them as an individual.

Thinking can be disrupted because the person is unable to selectively filter unimportant or extraneous information. The resultant expression of these thoughts is often vague or totally incomprehensible. Some sufferers experience blocking of their thoughts or thought withdrawal by an external agent. Mood is typically shallow or incongruous and individuals can experience loss of interest and social withdrawal.

Key point ▶

> Psychosis is a syndrome that includes the symptoms of delusions, hallucinations and disorganised speech and behaviour.

The World Health Organization's International Classification of Diseases, 10th edition (ICD-10) describes several subtypes of schizophrenia based on the symptom patterns that have been observed. These include paranoid, simple, hebephrenic and catatonic. **Paranoid schizophrenia**, the most common form, is marked by sudden onset, with prominent hallucinations and delusions, particularly of a persecutory nature. Those presenting predominantly with deterioration in personality, blunted affect and emotional and social withdrawal are diagnosed with **simple schizophrenia**. **Hebephrenia** is characterised by its insidious onset in adolescence with disturbances of thinking, perception, affect and behaviour. **Catatonic schizophrenia**, rarely seen today, involves disturbances of movement. These motor symptoms include increased muscle tone whereby the patient adopts unusual postures, which can be maintained for hours.

◀ *Key point*

> The four subtypes of schizophrenia are paranoid, simple, hebephrenic and catatonic.

The symptoms of schizophrenia can be categorised as being positive or negative, a concept introduced by Strauss *et al.* in 1974 (Table 5.1).

Positive symptoms	Negative symptoms
Hallucinations	Social withdrawal
Delusions	Avolition/apathy
Inappropriate affect	Blunted affect
Abnormalities of thought	Thought blocking
Agitation/excitement	Poverty of speech

Table 5.1

Symptoms of schizophrenia.

Positive symptoms

Positive symptoms include hallucinations, delusions, abnormalities of thought, inappropriate affect and agitation/excitement. They are often found in people in the acute phases of the illness and seem to reflect an excess of normal functions. They represent the presence in an individual of a behaviour that is not normally encountered.

Hallucinations are false perceptions in any of the senses: that is, the person perceives something for which there is no external stimulus. Schizophrenics will often hear voices talking about them, known as third-person auditory hallucinations, or hear voices in the second person commanding them to do something. Others report hearing their own thoughts being spoken back to them, a phenomenon known as thought echo. For the sufferer the voices seem very real. They can be loud and shouting, or sometimes just a whisper. They can be tolerable but for many the voices are distressing. They can intimidate the person, or be threatening and abusive. Many people with schizophrenia describe the voices as coming from behind them, through the walls, or from the television or radio.

Du Feu and McKenna (1999) investigated the experience of auditory hallucinations in the profoundly deaf. They found that deaf people describe auditory hallucinations in much the same way as those with normal hearing. They postulate that hallucinations are a non-perceptual abnormality that the patient interprets as perceptual. In other words, auditory hallucinations result from an abnormality affecting inner speech whereby the individual fails to recognise their inner speech for what it is. Brain scans of people who hear voices have found that when the person is experiencing hearing voices there is activity in the area of the brain that normally indicates that they are speaking. Auditory hallucinations can thus be described as, literally, inner speech.

Olfactory (smell), gustatory (taste) and tactile (touch) hallucinations are often misinterpreted as being caused by the acts of others. Visual (sight) hallucinations are less common.

Key point ▶

> Hallucinations are false perceptions in any of the senses. Auditory hallucinations are most commonly experienced in people with schizophrenia.

Delusions are strongly held false beliefs that have no basis in reality and that are at odds with the commonly held beliefs of others of the same culture. They tend to dominate the affected person's thoughts and often form as a consequence of trying to make sense of other symptoms. Delusions of control, influence or passivity often occur together. In this instance the patient may feel that s/he is under the control of another person or force and has no free will.

Other delusions often associated with schizophrenia include delusions of persecution, when patients believes that others are conspiring against them, or they may feel that events or the actions or words or others have special significance for them, feelings known as delusions of reference. Some experience persistent delusions of other kinds, such as religious or political identity, or extraordinary powers that are culturally inappropriate. For example, 'I am Jesus' or 'I can communicate with aliens and control the world' are beliefs often expressed by patients with schizophrenia.

Defining delusions can be difficult, however. Most people would not consider that believing yourself to be in touch with God is necessarily a delusion. Jones (1999) has identified several characteristics of delusions that help distinguish them from other strongly held beliefs, such as religious beliefs. Delusions form quickly and without great thought, and do not involve the imagination, whereas religious beliefs are usually arrived at gradually and involve much use of the imagination.

Key point ▶

> Delusions are strongly held false beliefs which have no basis in reality and which are at odds with the commonly held beliefs of others of the same culture.

Abnormalities of thought in a person with schizophrenia may produce **pressure of speech** as the individual attempts to express his/her rapidly forming thoughts and ideas. The association between these ideas can also be affected, producing jumbled, incoherent sentences. Words may be invented, a phenomenon known as neology, or used in unusual ways. People with a diagnosis of schizophrenia may also respond to situations in an emotionally inappropriate way, becoming excited when sobriety is required or showing sadness at a happy event.

Negative symptoms

The negative symptoms of schizophrenia, considered to be a reduction or loss of normal functions, include apathy, social withdrawal, poverty of thought, thought blocking and blunted affect, and are more often seen in people with chronic illness. They represent the absence of behaviour that is usually present in an individual. Pessimism and subjective sadness are not considered to be negative symptoms.

The person with negative symptoms may become unmotivated, losing the volition to engage in social activities, and slide into self-neglect. Washing, dressing and other basic needs are disregarded. The person's affect, the feeling experienced in connection with mood, may become blunted and s/he will appear to be emotionally flat. The person's conversation becomes limited and lacks the support of appropriate non-verbal communication. Poverty of thought and thought blocking lead to slow expression of ideas or abrupt pauses in conversation, as the person's mind appears to go blank. The negative symptoms of schizophrenia have been categorised as being either primary (transient or enduring) or secondary (to positive symptoms or antipsychotic drugs; Carpenter 1996).

> The negative symptoms of schizophrenia are considered to be a reduction or loss of normal functions.

◀ **Key point**

AETIOLOGY OF SCHIZOPHRENIA

Psychoses were once differentiated according to whether they were functional or organic in origin, a concept first introduced by Kraepelin (1919). Organic psychosis is brought about by some physical change in brain structure, whereas functional psychosis is a disorder of function rather than structure. Schizophrenia was seen as a functional psychotic disorder until technological advances in neuroimaging led researchers towards an organic basis for some forms of the illness. Improved levels of resolution, alongside functional imaging capabilities, is likely to lead researchers towards establishing a better understanding of the relationship between brain anatomy and function. The evidence thus far suggests that schizophrenia has a pathology associated with changes in the neural circuitry in key areas of the brain, rather than a neurodegenerative process.

The suspected link between schizophrenia and cigarette smoking is receiving increased interest. It has long been recognised that people with schizophrenia tend to smoke to excess. In fact, the rate of smoking in people with schizophrenia is two to three times that in the general population (Hughes *et al.*, 1986). The majority of those who smoke started smoking prior to the onset of their illness (Kelly and McCreadie, 1999). This raises the question: why do patients with schizophrenia smoke? There may be aspects of the illness that increase smoking in this group. Smoking may also act as an aetiological risk factor for schizophrenia (Kelly and McCreadie, 1999). Finally, genetic and/or environmental factors might predispose these patients to develop both schizophrenia and nicotine addiction (Maier and Schwab, 1998; Clarke, 1998).

Despite the accumulation of evidence, no specific causal agent has been identified for schizophrenia. Much of the research into the disorder is studying risk factors such as heredity, altered brain development and chemical imbalance. These will be examined in turn.

Key point ▶

> Risk factors for schizophrenia include heredity, altered brain development and chemical imbalance.

Genetics

There is strong evidence for a genetic component in the aetiology of schizophrenia. The lifetime risk of schizophrenia in first-degree relatives of affected probands is approximately 15%, a figure corresponding to 10 times the risk in the general population worldwide (Gottesman, 1991; Table 5.2). The presence of a genetic contribution to schizophrenia is given further credence by twin and adoption studies. Concordance rates for schizophrenia in monozygotic twins average 46%, compared to about 10% in dizygotic twins (McGuffin *et al.*, 1994), indicating that the higher the proportion of genetic material shared by the twins the greater the chance of developing the illness.

Key point ▶

> The higher the proportion of genetic material shared by a relative of someone with schizophrenia, the greater the chance of them developing the illness.

Studying the offspring of twins discordant for schizophrenia indicates that having a parent who is vulnerable to the illness is a significant risk factor irrespective of whether the parent actually has schizophrenia. The morbidity in the offspring of monozygotic twins discordant for the illness is the same, and is similar to that seen in the offspring of affected dizygotic twins. However, a much lower rate is seen in the offspring of the dizygotic twin who does not have the illness.

Table 5.2

Lifetime risk of developing schizophrenia (Gottesman, 1991).

Relationship to a person suffering from schizophrenia	Risk of suffering from schizophrenia (%)
Grandchild	5
Half-sibling	6
Sibling	9
Child of one schizophrenic parent	13
Child of two schizophrenic parents	46
Non-identical co-twin of a schizophrenic	17
Identical co-twin of a schizophrenic	48

Adoption studies indicate significantly higher rates of schizophrenia in biological relatives of affected individuals compared to adoptive relatives (Farmer *et al.*, 1987). Crow (1993) describes schizophrenia as one extreme on a psychosis continuum. Shared genetic material in relatives of people with schizophrenia may explain why they have some non-psychotic features that correlate with characteristics in the affected individual.

The mechanism of genetic inheritance is not clear, although a polygenic mode of transmission is likely. The combined action of these genes is hypothesised to produce vulnerability in the individual. The significant discordance between monozygotic twins implies that other factors must be present before this vulnerability manifests as illness. In other words, a predisposition to the disorder is inherited rather than the illness itself.

The interrelationship between genetic vulnerability and other aetiological factors forms the basis of the two-hit hypothesis: the development of schizophrenia not only requires the individual to have a genetic vulnerability, the first hit, but a second hit must also be sustained by way of the environment (Lieberman 1998). This hypothesis can be applied to other psychiatric disorders, although the genetic loading in schizophrenia seems to be higher than that postulated for other disorders.

A predisposition to schizophrenia is inherited, rather than the disorder itself.

◀ **Key point**

Despite a great deal of research in this area, the location and identification of genes predisposing individuals to schizophrenia has so far been generally unsuccessful. This is probably because inheritance of the predisposition is complex and because multiple genes with relatively small effects are operating. A number of approaches have been developed to try to resolve this situation, including linkage and anticipation studies. Linkage studies involve the use of genetic markers to attempt to locate the disease gene. Anticipation is a phenomenon seen in a number of single-gene disorders, such as Huntington's disease, in which unstable trinucleotide repeat sequences occur close to the disease genes. Claims that the first schizophrenia gene has been identified are soon to be reported in *Molecular Psychiatry*. German researchers working in the Department of Psychiatry and Psychotherapy at the Julius Maximilian's University in Würzburg believe that they have found a gene mutation on chromosome 22 that is in part responsible for the development of catatonic schizophrenia. However, the data were collected from a single large family and must be treated with caution.

The genetic liability for schizophrenia is likely to produce a multitude of clinical manifestations. Therefore, the risk to relatives of those with schizophrenia is not limited to schizophrenia alone. A study by Farmer *et al.* (1987) found much higher monozygotic/dizygotic concordance ratios when diagnoses such as schizotypal personality disorder and atypical psychosis were included alongside schizophrenia. The case is given further credence by Maier *et al.* (1992), who found that relatives of people with illnesses such as schizoaffective disorder are also significantly predisposed to schizophrenia. However, this predisposition is not generalised to all psychiatric disorders, suggesting that schizophrenia is only one possible outcome of increased liability.

The probability of developing schizophrenia may be influenced by the interaction of the genome with the environment. However, adoption away from a family in which schizophrenia is present does not reduce the risk to the adoptee. Time of onset may also suggest an environmental influence, although when schizophrenia occurs in two siblings it does so when they are of similar age rather than at the time of a shared experience (Crow and Done, 1986).

Assertions about the influence of environmental variance are generally made without valid measurement of the environment. There is an assumption that the environmental influences for monozygotic and dizygotic twins are similar. However, if monozygotic twins believe they are inherently more similar to each other than dizygotic twins, and their experiences as such are more closely linked, the assumption is flawed.

Neurodevelopment

There is growing evidence suggesting a role for structural and functional abnormalities of the brain in the aetiology of schizophrenia (Crow 1980). It is possible that neurodevelopmental disruption at the early stages of brain development *in utero* may later manifest as symptoms of the disorder. Deviances in the brains of people with schizophrenia at both the microscopic and macroscopic levels can be found compared to those of healthy individuals (Marsh *et al.*, 1994; Roberts *et al.*, 1993). Cellular positioning abnormalities consistent with genetic or teratogenic disturbances during gestation have been reported. Structural differences such as ventricular enlargement and temporal lobe reduction are seen in neuroimaging studies at both the onset and later stages of the illness, indicating that abnormalities are present at least as early as the onset of psychosis. Such differences are not confined to a subgroup but are characteristic of the group of patients with schizophrenia as a whole (Daniel *et al.*, 1991). Other studies suggest that the brains of people with schizophrenia are slightly smaller than those of non-affected individuals (Selemon *et al.*, 1995).

Obstetric complications such as perinatal hypoxia, viral infection and even Rhesus incompatibility may adversely impact fetal neurodevelopment, leading to the development of schizophrenia later in life. People born in the winter months are about 10% more likely to develop the illness, suggesting the involvement of seasonal environmental factors such as temperature or viral infection. There is evidence of a link between pregnancy and childbirth complications and the later development of schizophrenia in males (Hultman *et al.*, 1999). A team of scientists found that the development of schizophrenia is associated with underweight fetuses and suggest that reduced placental function may impair brain development, leading to increased vulnerability to later schizophrenia. The link for female children is weaker.

Children who later go on to develop schizophrenia have been observed to have neurobehavioural and neuromotor abnormalities. A study by Jones *et al.* (1994) highlighted various factors in children that were associated with later schizophrenia. These included delayed psychomotor milestones, speech problems, poorer educational test scores, social isolation and greater anxiety.

> There is growing evidence suggesting a role for structural and functional abnormalities of the brain in the aetiology of schizophrenia.

◀ *Key point*

Research into brain abnormalities in schizophrenia has yet to prove a neurodevelopmental origin for the expression of the illness. It may still be appropriate to view schizophrenia as a neurodegenerative condition, as hypothesised by Kraepelin (1919), with the progressive disease process at least partially active before the first overt symptoms of psychosis are evident. However, a neurodevelopmental approach may explain why the aetiology of schizophrenia has yet to be identified (Cannon and Mednick, 1991). Neurodevelopment follows a complex sequence of events that is far from being fully understood. Insults to the brain during its development will directly affect the resulting condition, producing a multitude of clinical manifestations. The nature of neurodevelopment, which continues throughout childhood, may also explain why the formal symptoms of schizophrenia are not seen until late adolescence or early adulthood (Weinberger, 1987). Bogerts (1989) suggests that the hormonal changes occurring at puberty influence already compromised limbic structures, resulting in psychotic symptomatology. Furthermore, unique individual experiences will interact with specific neuropathology, contributing further to the divergence of clinical presentations.

Neurochemistry

The many and varied symptoms of schizophrenia can be explained by a disturbance of neurochemical function, a plausible mode of expression of a genetic fault or altered brain development. The link between neurotransmitter disturbance and psychosis was first made following the synthesis of lysergic acid diethylamide (LSD) and its widespread illicit use. This drug produced symptoms of psychosis that were previously only seen in disorders such as schizophrenia. With the introduction of antipsychotic drugs in the 1950s, what emerged was a hypothesis that a functional excess of the neurotransmitter dopamine produces the positive symptoms of schizophrenia.

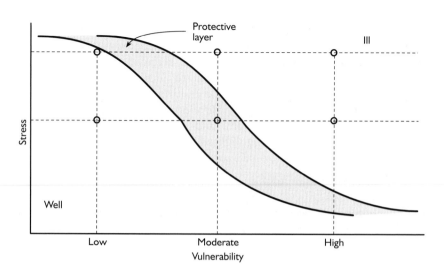

Figure 5.2

Stress-vulnerability model of mental illness

Key point ▶

> The many and varied symptoms of schizophrenia can be explained by a disturbance of neurochemical function.

It is widely recognised that schizophrenia is adversely affected by stress. The onset of the illness and relapses are often preceded by personal stressful events. These experiences, when they exceed the threshold of tolerance to the stress, produce overt symptoms of illness. The same experience in individuals who have higher levels of stress tolerance does not result in illness. This forms the basis of the stress-vulnerability hypothesis (Figure 5.2).

PHARMACOLOGICAL TREATMENT

There is increasing evidence for the need for early treatment of the symptoms of schizophrenia. A large study examining the course of the disorder between onset and initial treatment (Hafner *et al.*, 1999) makes a good case for early detection and treatment in schizophrenia. The authors suggest that considerable social impairment may occur during the prodrome and the first onset of psychotic symptoms. Delaying treatment is associated with longer spells of illness and increased likelihood of progressive deterioration (Lieberman *et al.*, 1993). The response to antipsychotic medication also seems to change over time. The treatment of first-episode patients seems to produce the most favourable response, while the response to antipsychotics tends to decline as patients have further episodes of illness. Other studies conclude that there is an increased risk of relapse following abrupt cessation of antipsychotic treatment compared with gradual withdrawal. Kissling *et al.* (1991) advocate continued treatment with antipsychotics for 1-2 years following a first psychotic episode and at least 5 years for patients who have had several episodes. The rate of relapse in the first couple of years is significantly higher for those individuals who stop treatment during this time.

> Delaying treatment for schizophrenia is associated with longer spells of illness and increased likelihood of progressive deterioration.

Pharmacodynamics

The pharmacological treatment of schizophrenia using antipsychotic drugs requires an understanding of four key neurotransmitter systems in the central nervous system: dopamine, serotonin (5-hydroxytryptamine, 5-HT), acetylcholine and glutamate.

> The pharmacological treatment of schizophrenia requires an understanding of four key neurotransmitter systems: dopamine, serotonin (5-hydroxytryptamine, 5-HT), acetylcholine and glutamate.

Dopamine

Dopamine is produced in dopaminergic neurones before its release into the synapse. In the synapse it is able to bind with a multitude of dopamine receptors, the most significant being the dopamine-2 (D_2) receptor, before its removal to the presynaptic neurone by a dopamine transporter. Four dopamine pathways in the brain explain both the antipsychotic action of drugs and their adverse effects (Figure 5.3). The mesolimbic dopamine pathway projects from the midbrain to an area of the limbic system that is involved in producing the symptoms of psychosis (i.e. delusions and hallucinations). A similar pathway is the mesocortical dopamine pathway, which also projects from the midbrain.

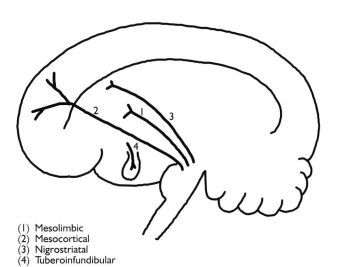

Figure 5.3

Dopamine pathways

(1) Mesolimbic
(2) Mesocortical
(3) Nigrostriatal
(4) Tuberoinfundibular

This pathway terminates in the limbic cortex and is postulated to have a role in mediating positive and negative symptoms of psychosis, or possibly in producing the neuroleptic-induced deficit syndrome. The nigrostriatal dopamine pathway projects from the substantia nigra to the basal ganglia and is involved in the co-ordination of movement. The final pathway, the tuberoinfundibular dopamine pathway, projects from the hypothalamus to the anterior pituitary gland, where it controls the release of prolactin.

Key point ▶

> Four dopamine pathways in the brain, the mesolimbic, mesocortical, nigrostriatal and tuberoinfundibular pathways, explain both the antipsychotic action of drugs and their adverse effects.

Serotonin

Serotonin is produced in serotoninergic neurones from the amino acid precursor tryptophan. When released into the synapse it binds with both presynaptic and postsynaptic serotonin receptors, before its removal to the presynaptic neurone by a serotonin-selective transport pump. Several serotonin pathways emanating from the midbrain are hypothesised to account for the actions of serotonin. Projections to the prefrontal cortex may mediate its cognitive effects. Other pathways are thought to be involved with the actions of antidepressant and anxiolytic drugs, and in the treatment of obsessive–compulsive disorder (OCD) and eating disorders. Of particular interest are the serotonin

Figure 5.4

Inhibition of dopamine release by serotonin in the nigrostriatal dopamine pathway

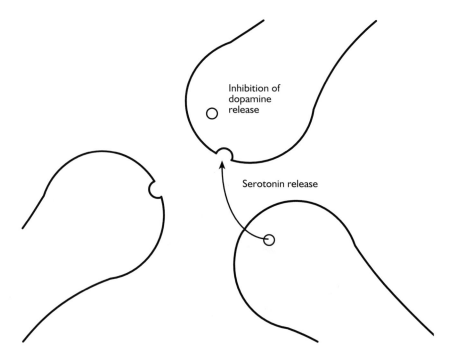

Inhibition of
dopamine
release

Serotonin release

pathways that make connections with dopamine neurones in the nigros-triatal and tuberoinfundibular pathways. The action of serotonin on the dopamine neurones is to cause the inhibition of dopamine release (Figure 5.4).

Serotonin acts to inhibit the release of dopamine.

◀ **Key point**

Acetylcholine

Acetylcholine is a neurotransmitter produced and released by choli-nergic neurones. The acetylcholine receptors are numerous and are generally divided into nicotinic and muscarinic cholinergic receptors. The muscarinic subtype is responsible for mediating the side-effects of anticholinergic drugs, including dry mouth, blurred vision, constipation and urinary retention. Muscarinic receptors are also thought to be involved in memory. The significance of acetylcholine is apparent in its relationship with dopamine in the nigrostriatal dopamine pathway. Dopamine neurones, through their postsynaptic connections with choli-nergic neurones, are responsible for the suppression of cholinergic activity (Figure 5.5).

Dopamine neurones are responsible for the suppression of choli-nergic activity.

◀ **Key point**

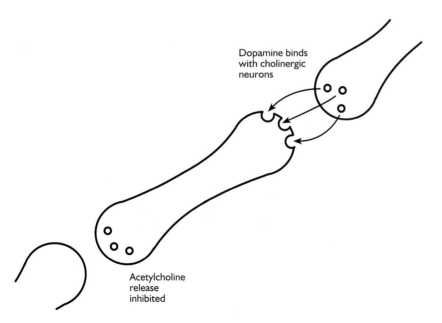

Dopamine binds
with cholinergic
neurons

Acetylcholine
release
inhibited

Figure 5.5

Relationship between dopamine and acetylcholine in the nigrostriatal dopamine pathway

Glutamate

The final key neurotransmitter system involves glutamate. Glutamate mediates its actions at a ligand-gated calcium ion channel, producing a fast, excitatory response. It is hypothesised that an excitotoxic mechanism involving glutamate may be responsible for the neurodegeneration seen in schizophrenia and possibly other neurodegenerative disorders such as Alzheimer's, Huntington's and Parkinson's diseases. The process seems to involve an overactivity of the glutamate system causing an influx of calcium into the neurone. It is the presence of too much calcium that stimulates intracellular enzymes to produce free radicals, chemicals that ultimately lead to cell death. Glutamate antagonists can provide neuroprotection by blocking the neurotransmission that leads to the excitotoxicity. Alternatively, free radical scavengers can provide protection by removal of the free radicals that lead to cell death. Vitamin E is currently being trialled for this purpose.

Key point ▶

An excitotoxic mechanism involving glutamate may be responsible for the neurodegeneration seen in schizophrenia.

In order to appreciate the pharmacological treatment of schizophrenia, it is important to remember the pathology of the symptoms produced by the illness. As detailed above, the symptoms are generally categorised as either positive or negative, but also include symptoms associated with cognition and emotion. The dopamine hypothesis (Matthysee, 1977), a neurochemical explanation for schizophrenia, states that an excess of dopamine activity in the mesolimbic dopamine pathway produces the positive symptoms of psychosis (delusions, hallucinations, disorganised speech and behaviour). The negative symptoms (emotional and social withdrawal, blunted affect, avolition (lack of 'drive'), anhedonia, alogia (impaired logical thinking) and passivity), on the other hand, may be produced by a deficiency of dopamine neurotransmission in the mesocortical pathway.

The conventional antipsychotic drugs share the ability to block dopamine-2 receptors. They are also able to block histamine, muscarinic/cholinergic and alpha-1-adrenergic receptors to varying degrees, but tend to lack the ability to block serotonin receptors, a feature of the new atypical antipsychotics. This divergence produces the variation in the side-effect profiles of these drugs, with some being more sedative (e.g. chlorpromazine), some having a high propensity to produce extrapyramidal side-effects (EPSEs; e.g. haloperidol) and others having greater cardiotoxicity (e.g. thioridazine). There is little discernible difference between the therapeutic efficacy of the conventional antipsychotics.

It is important that practitioners recognise the difference between non-specific sedation and antipsychotic effect. If sedation is required as part of the treatment plan, this should be provided by a recognised sedative such as a benzodiazepine. This can be withdrawn when it is no longer necessary and does not carry the risks associated with high doses of antipsychotic medication.

The conventional antipsychotics share the ability to block dopamine-2 receptors, but lack the ability to block serotonin receptors, a feature of the new atypical antipsychotics.

◀ **Key point**

While the conventional antipsychotics have proven efficacy in reducing the positive symptoms of psychosis, they are also capable of producing extrapyramidal side-effects and tardive dyskinesia. These effects, both positive and negative, are a result of the drugs' ability to block dopamine-2 receptors. The therapeutic effects are produced by blockade in the mesolimbic dopamine pathway. The conventional antipsychotics are not selective for this pathway and will block dopamine-2 receptors in all areas of the brain. Blockade in the nigrostriatal dopamine pathway, which projects to a part of the extrapyramidal system, the basal ganglia, produces extrapyramidal side-effects. These side-effects are significant and include dystonias, pseudoparkinsonism, akathisia (described below) and dysphoria (a state of mental unease).

Extrapyramidal side-effects are the result of a drug-induced imbalance between dopamine and acetylcholine in the nigrostriatal dopamine pathway. Ordinarily, dopamine released from dopaminergic neurones suppresses the release of acetylcholine from the cholinergic neurones in the pathway. Conventional antipsychotics block the dopamine receptors in the postsynaptic cholinergic neurones, thereby releasing the brake on acetylcholine activity. This elevated activity is responsible for the production of the extrapyramidal side-effects. Anticholinergics, such as procyclidine, are useful in the treatment of dystonias and pseudoparkinsonism. They work by competing for the cholinergic/muscarinic receptors. Akathisia, an inner state of restlessness that has been linked to aggression and suicidality, often benefits from treatment with propranolol.

Persistent antagonism of dopamine receptors in the nigrostriatal pathway may produce a proliferation of receptors as the neurones attempt to counteract this blockade. This is sometimes seen in long-term treatment with conventional antipsychotics, producing a hyperkinetic movement disorder known as **tardive dyskinesia**. This is a serious and potentially irreversible adverse effect that results in involuntary movements, particularly in the face and trunk. Facial grimacing, jaw and tongue movements and gyrating hip movements are often obvious and stigmatising.

The incidence of tardive dyskinesia increases with duration and dosage of antipsychotic treatment and is thought to be in excess of 50% among patients on long-term conventional antipsychotic medication. Prevention, the main form of treatment, includes the use of low doses of drugs for the shortest possible time. Antipsychotics that are less likely to cause tardive dyskinesia are preferable and the need for anticholinergics should be regularly reassessed.

While anticholinergics worsen existing tardive dyskinesia, there is little evidence for anticholinergics being an independent risk factor. If tardive dyskinesia develops anticholinergics should be withdrawn and, if appropriate, the antipsychotic should be slowly withdrawn or changed to a more suitable drug such as clozapine or olanzapine. All patients taking antipsychotic medication should be regularly assessed for the presence of abnormal involuntary body movements using a scale such as the Abnormal Involuntary Movement Scale (AIMS; Munetz and Benjamin, 1988).

It is worth noting that tardive dyskinesia can occur in untreated schizophrenia. This implies that antipsychotics are not the only risk factor for the development of the condition.

Key point ▶

> Extrapyramidal side effects, including dystonias, pseudoparkinsonism, akathisia and dysphoria, are the result of a drug-induced imbalance between dopamine and acetylcholine in the nigrostriatal pathway.

The mesocortical dopamine pathway, closely associated with the mesolimbic dopamine pathway, is thought to have a role in mediating positive and negative symptoms of psychosis. The conventional antipsychotics are thought to produce secondary negative symptoms by suppressing dopamine activity in the mesocortical dopamine pathway. Primary negative symptoms are most responsive to pharmacological treatment during the acute phase of the illness, and become less responsive as the illness progresses. Wyatt (1995) found that early intervention with antipsychotics improves the prognosis for schizophrenia and may reduce the likelihood of developing enduring negative symptoms.

Key point ▶

> The mesocortical pathway is thought to have a role in mediating positive and negative symptoms of psychosis.

A further pathway adversely affected by the conventional antipsychotics is the tuberoinfundibular dopamine pathway. This short pathway links the hypothalamus with the anterior pituitary and controls the release of the hormone prolactin. Dopamine receptor antagonism in this pathway leads to an elevation of prolactin, a condition that can produce galactorrhoea (inappropriate lactation) in women.

Key point ▶

> The tuberoinfundibular pathway controls the release of the hormone prolactin.

The conventional antipsychotics have varying degrees of in-built anticholinergic activity and thereby have varying propensities to produce extrapyramidal side-effects. However, the blockade of cholinergic/muscarinic receptors produces its own set of side-effects. The anticholinergic side-effects are dry mouth, blurred vision, constipation and drowsiness. Further side-effects of the conventional antipsychotics include weight gain and drowsiness, produced by blockade of histamine receptors, and drowsiness, lowered blood pressure and dizziness produced by blockade of alpha-1-adrenergic receptors.

> Anticholinergic drugs have their own set of side effects, including dry mouth, blurred vision, constipation and drowsiness.

◀ **Key point**

The conventional antipsychotics have certain advantages over the newer atypical agents. They have comparable efficacy in terms of treating positive symptoms of psychosis compared with some of the atypicals, and are much cheaper. Many are also available in intramuscular forms for use in emergencies or as depots. However, the poor side-effect profile of the conventional drugs is leading to a reduction in their use as first-line treatments and, indeed, for long-term maintenance. It may still be acceptable to continue with conventional antipsychotics in patients who are stabilised and tolerating the side-effects, or as an alternative to the atypical antipsychotics when these have failed.

The atypical antipsychotics are so-named because of their lack of propensity to produce extrapyramidal side-effects or tardive dyskinesia. The term 'atypical' also tends to imply a reduced likelihood for increased prolactin levels and greater efficacy in the treatment of negative symptoms. It is these features that provide the distinction between the atypical and conventional antipsychotics. It is thought that these differences are the result of the different mechanism of action of the two groups of drugs. The atypical drugs are serotonin–dopamine antagonists (SDAs), compared with the conventional drugs, which lack serotonin antagonism.

> The atypical antipsychotics are serotonin–dopamine antagonists and are so-named because of their lack of propensity to produce extrapyramidal side-effects or tardive dyskinesia.

◀ **Key point**

Serotonin–dopamine antagonists block both serotonin-2A receptors and dopamine-2 receptors. The relationship between serotonin and dopamine in two dopamine pathways seems to be the key to the improved side-effect profile of these drugs. In the nigrostriatal dopamine pathway, serotonin inhibits the release of dopamine. It does this through its presynaptic interface with dopaminergic neurones. SDAs block both serotonin and dopamine receptors in this pathway. The effect is to allow an excessive release of dopamine, which effectively competes with the

SDA for the dopamine-2 receptors. This reversal of dopamine-2 blockade, less than 70% with the SDAs compared to approximately 90% with the conventional antipsychotics, reduces the likelihood of SDAs producing extrapyramidal symptoms or tardive dyskinesia.

A similar arrangement exists between serotonin and dopamine in the tuberoinfundibular dopamine pathway. The normal action of dopamine is to inhibit the secretion of prolactin from the anterior pituitary gland, while the normal action of serotonin is to stimulate prolactin secretion. Conventional antipsychotics are solely dopamine antagonists and therefore block dopamine receptors, thus promoting the release of prolactin. The consequence for women is the side-effect of galactorrhoea – milk production in someone who is neither pregnant nor has given birth. The effect of the SDAs, which also block serotonin, is to nullify the blockade of dopamine and thereby regain the *status quo*. The atypical antipsychotics thus have a much-reduced propensity to produce galactorrhoea.

Key point ▶

> The relationship between serotonin and dopamine in two dopamine pathways seems to be the key to the improved side-effect profile of the atypical antipsychotics compared with the conventional antipsychotics.

It is questionable whether atypical antipsychotics are more effective than the conventional antipsychotics in the treatment of the primary negative symptoms of schizophrenia. Undoubtedly, the atypicals treat the positive symptoms without concomitant production of secondary negative symptoms. It is hypothesised that primary negative symptoms result from a lack of dopamine activity in the mesocortical dopamine pathway, possibly due to excessive inhibition here by serotonin. The action of the SDAs is to block the serotonin receptors in this pathway, thus enhancing dopamine activity. Despite this, there is no evidence to support the contention that the atypical antipsychotics having greater efficacy than the conventional antipsychotics in the treatment of primary enduring negative symptoms.

The atypical antipsychotics are now widely recognised as being the treatment of choice for both the positive and negative symptoms of schizophrenia, both in terms of first-line treatment and long-term maintenance therapy. They have the benefit of a much improved side-effect profile and, while they are more expensive than the conventional antipsychotics, there is evidence that they are more cost-effective. The atypicals have been shown to produce better compliance and reduced risk of relapse and need for rehospitalisation.

Key point ▶

> Atypical antipsychotics are now widely recognised as being the treatment of choice for both the positive and negative symptoms of schizophrenia.

What gives the atypical antipsychotics improved efficacy? The answer seems to amount to more than their ability to block serotonin-2 and dopamine-2 receptors. The atypicals are antagonists for a wide range of serotonin and dopamine receptors, and act on cholinergic, noradrenergic and histaminic neurotransmitter systems. No longer is it the aim to find antipsychotics that are highly selective for a single neurotransmitter receptor. The enhanced efficacy of the atypical antipsychotics is probably due to their complex action at a multitude of receptor sites.

Treatment-resistant or **refractory schizophrenia** can be defined as a lack of response to two antipsychotics. The only drug that has unquestionable efficacy in the treatment of refractory schizophrenia is **clozapine** (Clozaril) It is debatable whether other drugs given the atypical label have any efficacy in refractory schizophrenia, despite an assumption by many clinicians that there is a link between the nonproduction of extrapyramidal side-effects and improved efficacy. Endless trials of other antipsychotics therefore seems pointless, particularly considering that the longer the period of uncontrolled symptoms the worse the prognosis. Studies have shown that response rates in excess of 60% can be achieved with clozapine if the drug is given for up to a year (Meltzer *et al.*, 1989).

Treatment-resistant schizophrenia can be defined as a lack of response to two antipsychotics.

◀ **Key point**

The initiation of clozapine treatment must be closely monitored and is restricted to patients who are registered with the Clozaril Patient Monitoring Service (CPMS). Treatment begins with an initial dose of 12.5 mg at night and the dose is gradually increased over a period of 2–3 weeks. A dose of around 400 mg/day is desirable, although there may be a need to increase this to a maximum of 900 mg/day. Increments of 50 mg/day every 2 weeks are typical.

A study by Meltzer *et al.* (1989) suggested that a delayed response to clozapine of up to 9 months is not uncommon, leading to a trial period of 1 year becoming the standard. Many clinicians now favour increasing the dose to its maximum over several weeks if no response is observed, allowing for an evaluation over 8 weeks at the maximum tolerated dose and then withdrawing the clozapine if there is still no response. This usually leads to a trial period of no more than 6 months (Conley *et al.*, 1997).

Once a desirable therapeutic benefit is achieved, many patients can be maintained on lower doses. This requires careful downward titration to a level of 150–300 mg/day. The termination of clozapine treatment should take the form of a gradual reduction in dose over a period of at least 1–2 weeks. Restarting treatment when there has been a break in treatment of more than 2 days necessitates returning to a daily dose of 12.5 mg. The rate of upward titration can be quicker than that recommended for initial treatment.

Treatment with clozapine carries certain risks. Approximately 4% of people taking clozapine develop a condition known as neutropenia, a fall in the number of neutrophils (white blood cells). This leaves the person vulnerable to infections and can, in rare cases, be fatal. The development of neutropenia does not seem to be dose-related, nor is duration of treatment a reliable indicator. The risks of neutropenia and the more advanced condition agranulocytosis are well managed by the CPMS. These are the only adverse effects likely to necessitate discontinuation of clozapine.

Key point ▶

> Approximately 4% of people taking clozapine develop a condition known as neutropenia, a fall in the number of neutrophils. This can develop into the potentially fatal condition agranulocytosis.

Other adverse effects associated with clozapine include drowsiness, hypotension and hypertension, weight gain, constipation, hypersalivation and seizures. The majority can be managed, although postural hypotension and weight gain are particularly troublesome. Reducing the dose of clozapine or slowing its titration manages hypotension best. Weight gain is very common and the early involvement of a dietitian is recommended.

Future treatments

Many herbal, nutritional and combination products are commonly being used as treatments for psychiatric conditions. They are readily available at pharmacies and are generally taken without informing a doctor. This raises concern, as there is a lack of knowledge about herb–drug and nutrient–drug interactions. Despite these concerns, there may be potential benefits for their use in the future treatment of schizophrenia. For example, neuronal membranes contain high proportions of several essential fatty acids. It has been suggested that depletion of omega-3 fatty acids impairs membrane function and may be of aetiological importance in schizophrenia and other psychiatric disorders (Hillbrand et al., 1997). Dietary supplementation could well become a complementary treatment of the future.

Key point ▶

> Dietary supplements, such as omega-3 fatty acids, could become a complementary future treatment for schizophrenia.

Pharmacokinetics

So far this chapter has dealt mainly with drug receptor interactions, the pharmacodynamics of antipsychotics. Another important aspect of psychopharmacology is pharmacokinetics – the way in which drugs move through the body. The cytochrome P450 enzyme systems are largely responsible for the way in which antipsychotics are absorbed, distributed, metabolised and finally excreted, and are worthy of consideration.

◄ **Key point**

> The cytochrome P450 enzyme systems are largely responsible for the way in which antipsychotics are absorbed, distributed, metabolised and finally excreted.

The cytochrome P450 enzymes number many, although not all of them are found in every individual. Their primary action is the transformation of drugs, either in the gut wall or in the liver, to a form that can be excreted from the body. **Clozapine** and **olanzapine** are drugs that are metabolised by the cytochrome P450 enzyme 1A2. **Fluvoxamine**, an antidepressant, inhibits 1A2. In the event of a person taking fluvoxamine alongside one of these atypical antipsychotics, the dose of the antipsychotic may need to be reduced to account for the lack of 1A2 activity. Smoking, however, has the reverse effect of increasing the activity of 1A2. The consequence for smokers, therefore, is the probable need for higher doses of clozapine or olanzapine compared with non-smokers. This is a particularly important consideration for patients who start smoking or increase their smoking.

The cytochrome P450 enzyme 2D6 also has metabolic functions relevant to psychopharmacology. It is responsible for metabolising clozapine, olanzapine and **risperidone**. The selective serotonin reuptake inhibitor (SSRI) class of antidepressants inhibits 2D6. The dose of clozapine and olanzapine, therefore, may need to be lowered when given concomitantly with an SSRI. The significance for risperidone is uncertain, as its metabolites are also active.

◄ **Key point**

> Smokers may need higher doses of clozapine or olanzapine compared with non-smokers. Conversely, the dose of clozapine or olanzapine may need to be reduced when given concomitantly with an SSRI.

Interactions with non-psychotropic drugs also require monitoring. The cytochrome P450 enzyme 3A4, which metabolises clozapine and **quetiapine** among others, although weakly inhibited by the antidepressants fluoxetine, fluvoxamine and nefazodone, is strongly inhibited by the antibiotic erythromycin. This is clinically significant and may require a reduction in the dose of the atypical antipsychotic.

Cytochrome P450 enzyme 3A4 is also affected by **carbamazepine**, a drug used to stabilise mood. Carbamazepine stimulates the enzyme to become more active over time. Since 3A4 is responsible for metabolising carbamazepine, this increased activity leads to a reduction in the level of carbamazepine. If carbamazepine is used concomitantly with clozapine or quetiapine, the dose of the antipsychotic may also need to be increased. Later withdrawal of carbamazepine may also require a reduction in the dose of the antipsychotic, since the effects of carbama-zepine on 3A4 subside with time.

Pharmacogenetics

Pharmacogenetics is the study of the link between positive and negative clinical responses to drugs and the specific genetic makeup of the patient. This will allow us to predict with greater certainty which patients would be most likely to benefit from treatment with a specific drug. It may also allow us to predict the likelihood of a better toler-ability of one drug compared to another. While still in its infancy, this approach has the potential to take away the trial-and-error associated with prescribing drugs for schizophrenia.

Key point ▶

> Pharmacogenetics may allow us to predict with greater certainty which patients would be most likely to benefit from treatment with a specific drug.

Treatment adherence

The value of treatment in schizophrenia is now widely accepted. Failure to adhere to established treatment regimens is clinically significant and is associated with an increased risk of relapse (Kissling, 1994) and rehos-pitalisation (Green, 1988). However, approximately 50% of people with a diagnosis of schizophrenia do not adhere to their medication regimen (Kane, 1985). This proportion is similar to that found in other chronic illnesses such as diabetes or hypertension (Ley, 1992). Repeated studies implicate poor adherence as an important factor in the length of readmissions and eventual outcome (Gaebel and Pietzcker, 1985; Verghese *et al.*, 1989; Helgason, 1990; Haywood *et al.*, 1995). Non-adherence has also been identified as being predictive of violent behaviour in patients with psychotic disorders (Fuller Torrey, 1994). Kissling (1994) argues that, with consistent relapse prevention, the rate of relapse in schizophrenia could be lowered to about 15% (currently half the number of patients diagnosed with schizophrenia relapse within the first year of remission, and about 85% do so within the first 5 years). Bebbington (1995) estimates the cost of non-adherence in the UK to be in excess of £100m.

Key point ▶

> Failure to adhere to established treatment regimens is clinically significant and is associated with an increased risk of relapse and rehospitalisation. However, approximately 50% of people with a diagnosis of schizophrenia do not adhere to their medication regimen.

The reasons for accepting or refusing treatment are extremely complex. Perceived side-effects, insight, health beliefs and elements of psychopathology have all been linked to adherence. The side-effects of medication are often regarded as contributing to non-adherence, although the findings of studies are contradictory. A study by Hoge *et al.* (1990) found that the use of anticholinergics improved adherence where extrapyramidal side-effects were a problem. It is feasible, therefore, that the introduction of the atypical antipsychotics, with their much reduced propensity to produce extrapyramidal side-effects, will lead to better adherence. It is important, however, to recognise the potential for the atypical antipsychotics to produce an array of other distressing side-effects, which may also influence adherence. Fleischhaker *et al.* (1994) stress the importance of recognising the significance of side-effects for patients by providing information and advice about the best ways to manage them should they arise. Hughes *et al.* (1997) suggest that the way patients view their side-effects has a greater impact on adherence than the mere presence of side-effects.

> Perceived side effects, insight, health beliefs and elements of psycho-pathology have all been linked to adherence.

◀ **Key point**

The relationship between adherence with treatment regimens and insight has been cited by many authors (Bartko *et al.*, 1988; McEvoy *et al.*, 1989; Buchanan, 1992; Kemp and Lambert 1995). Lack of insight is often cited as an important contributor to non-adherence (Bartko *et al.*, 1990). Sanz *et al.* (1998) found that there was a positive relationship between insight and adherence, with neither of these concepts being related to either overall psychopathology or to levels of cognitive performance. A study by Budd *et al.* (1996), however, failed to find a relationship between insight and adherence.

Health beliefs and attitudes may also influence a patient's adherence to treatment. Budd *et al.* (1996) found that health beliefs were more predictive of adherence than measures of insight. Hughes *et al.* (1997) argued that health beliefs were capable of explaining adherence in the severely mentally ill. They recognised, however, the difficulty of modifying health beliefs compared with some of the other factors that influence adherence.

There may also be a relationship between the presence of psychotic symptoms and levels of adherence. Kemp and David (1997) identify many positive symptoms thought to be associated with poor adherence. Negative symptoms and cognitive deficit may also contribute to poor adherence if the ability to understand the purpose of medication is impaired.

Many strategies have been employed to improve adherence with antipsychotics. Most of these have used an educational approach in the belief that, if people have a greater knowledge about their medication, they are more likely to take it as prescribed. Psychoeducation may be defined as a process leading to the education of patients suffering from severe mental illness about all aspects of the illness, its consequences and its treatment. The aim of the intervention, therefore, is to increase the patient's understanding of the illness, with the intended outcome of reducing non-adherence with treatment regimes and hence reducing relapse rates. Mikhail (1981) suggests that patients should be provided with information regarding the benefits of various health actions and helped to choose the action with the highest probability of success. Atkinson *et al.* (1996) advocate attendance at education groups. They believe that this can lead to significant gains in social functioning and quality of life without specific skills training. Gaebel (1997) argues that the use of educational tools to improve adherence should be generally enforced. A study by Macpherson *et al.* (1996), however, found that patient education led to no change in adherence. Boczkowski *et al.* (1985) demonstrated that adherence changed minimally with psychoeducation, whereas behavioural approaches led to significantly better adherence. They compared the effects of a behavioural-tailoring and a psychoeducational intervention in outpatients with chronic schizophrenia. Follow-up after 3 months showed that the behavioural-tailoring group were significantly more adherent. The behavioural-tailoring intervention included practical guidelines, such as stimulus cues to facilitate remembering, and self-monitoring calendars. The psychoeducational intervention consisted of didactic information on the illness and reasons for taking medication.

Education programmes also have to consider the maintenance of gains made. Streicker *et al.* (1986) found that initial improvements in attitudes decayed over time. This suggests the need for booster sessions to consolidate any gains made. Corrigan *et al.* (1990) have highlighted the need for greater collaboration in attempts to tackle adherence. Barriers to partnership in treatment include poor clinician–patient relationships and difficulties with treatment delivery systems.

Kemp *et al.* (1996) have developed a 'compliance therapy' intervention based on a self-regulatory systems approach, which takes into account the congruence between patient and practitioner with respect to illness representation, coping behaviour and appraisal of action. Patients are encouraged to take an active role in illness monitoring and negotiating treatment decisions in partnership with mental health professionals. 'Compliance therapy' draws on motivational interviewing principles and cognitive–behavioural approaches, and has been found to improve adherence, attitudes to treatment, insight and global functioning in people with a diagnosis of schizophrenia. Motivational interviewing is a technique that has been successfully used with ambivalent groups and has been adapted to take a more therapeutic stance for those with severe mental illness. Cognitive-behavioural approaches include the use of normalisation, and addressing specific psychotic symptoms, if they impinge on adherence. An 18-month follow-up to this study concluded that 'compliance therapy' could improve survival in the community after an acute psychotic episode (Kemp *et al.*, 1998).

TESTS TO AID DIAGNOSIS

A team of scientists have conducted a study using brain-imaging techniques to recognise substantial changes in brain structure, which appear to take place before the onset of psychotic symptoms (Fannon *et al.*, 2000). The study also raises the possibility that new treatments could be developed to halt the progression of the illness. Wyatt (1991) found that earlier treatment with medication was associated with better long-term prognosis. Another test, which measures the way people blink in response to being startled by a loud noise, may highlight a vulnerability marker in a subset of people with schizophrenia (Crawford *et al.*, 1998). Diagnosis in schizophrenia may also be enhanced by simple blood and breath tests in the future.

SUMMARY

This chapter has given a clinical picture of schizophrenia and addressed the neurodevelopmental and neurodegenerative hypotheses for the disorder. The major dopamine pathways have been considered in relation to the dopamine hypothesis of schizophrenia and the pharmacodynamics and pharmacokinetics of antipsychotic drugs were discussed. Diagnostic tests and treatment adherence have been introduced.

REFERENCES AND FURTHER READING

Atkinson, J.M., Coia, D.A., Gilmour, W.H. and Harper, J.P. (1996) The impact of education groups for people with schizophrenia on social functioning and quality of life. *British Journal of Psychiatry*, **168**, 199–204.

Bartko, G., Herceg, I. and Zador, G. (1988) Clinical symptomatology and drug compliance in schizophrenic patients. *Acta Psychiatrica Scandinavica*, **77**, 74–76.

Bartko, G., Frecska, E., Horvath, S. *et al.* (1990) Predicting neuroleptic response from a combination of multilevel variables in acute schizophrenic patients. *Acta Psychiatrica Scandinavica*, **82**, 408–412.

Bebbington, P.E. (1995) The content and context of compliance. *International Clinical Psychopharmacology*, **9**(Suppl. 5): 41–50.

Boczkowski, J.A., Zeichner, A. and Desanto, N. (1985) Neuroleptic compliance among chronic schizophrenic patients. *Journal of Consulting and Clinical Psychology*, **53**, 666–671.

Bogerts, B. (1989) Limbic and paralimbic pathology in schizophrenia: Interaction with age and stress related factors. In: *Schizophrenia: Scientific Progress* (ed. S.C. Schulz and C.A. Tamminga). Oxford University Press, Oxford, pp. 216–226

Buchanan, A. (1992) A two-year prospective study of treatment compliance in patients with schizophrenia. *Psychological Medicine*, **22**, 787–797.

Budd, R.J., Hughes, I.C.T. and Smith, J.A. (1996) Health beliefs and compliance with antipsychotic medication. *British Journal of Clinical Psychology*, **35**, 393–397.

Caldwell, C.B. and Gottesman, I.I. (1992) Schizophrenia, a high risk factor for suicide: clues to risk reduction. *Suicide and Life Threatening Behaviour*, **22**, 479–493.

Cannon, T.D. and Mednick, S.A. (1991) Fetal neural development and adult schizophrenia: an elaboration of the paradigm. In: *Fetal Neural Development and Adult Schizophrenia* (ed. S.A. Mednick, T.D. Cannon, C.E. Barr and M. Lyon). Cambridge University Press, Cambridge, pp. 227–237.

Carpenter, W.T. (1996) The treatment of negative symptoms: pharmacological and methodological issues. *British Journal of Psychiatry*, **168**(Suppl. 29), 17–22.

Castle, D.J., Abel, K., Takei, N. and Murray, R.M. (1995) Gender differences in schizophrenia: hormonal effect or subtypes. *Schizophrenia Bulletin*, **21**, 1–12.

Clarke, P.B.S. (1998) Tobacco smoking, genes and dopamine. *Lancet*, **353**, 84–85.

Conley, R.R., Carpenter, W.T. and Tamminga, C.A. (1997) Time to clozapine response in a standardised trial. *American Journal of Psychiatry*, **154**, 1243–1247.

Corrigan, P.W., Liberman, R.P. and Engel, J.D. (1990) From non-compliance to collaboration in the treatment of schizophrenia. *Hospital and Community Psychiatry*, **41**, 1203–1211.

Crawford, T.J., Sharma, B.K., Puri, R.M. *et al.* (1998) Saccadic eye movements in families multiply affected with schizophrenia: the Maudsley family study. *American Journal of Psychiatry*, **155**, 1703–1710.

Crow, T.J. (1980) Molecular pathology of schizophrenia: more than one disease process? *British Medical Journal*, **280**, 66–68.

Crow, T.J. (1993) Schizophrenia: diagnostic boundaries, epidemiology and brain changes. *The Clinician*, **11**, 2–17.

Crow, T.J. and Done, D.J. (1986) Age of onset of schizophrenia in siblings: a test of the contagion hypothesis. *Psychiatry Research*, **18**, 107–117.

Daniel, D.G., Goldberg, T.E., Gibbons, R.D. and Weinberger, D.R. (1991) Lack of bimodal distribution of ventricular size in schizophrenia: a Gaussian mixture analysis of 1056 cases and controls. *Biological Psychiatry*, **30**, 887–903.

Fannon, D., Chitnis, X., Doku, V. *et al.* (2000) Features of structural brain abnormality detected in first-episode psychosis. *American Journal of Psychiatry*, **157**, 1829–1834.

Farmer, A.E., McGuffin, P. and Gottesman, I.I. (1987) Twin concordance for DSM-III schizophrenia. *Archives of General Psychiatry*, **44**, 634–641.

Du Feu, M. and McKenna, P.J. (1999) Profoundly deaf patients do hear voices. *Acta Psychiatrica Scandinavica*, **99**, 453–459.

Fleischhaker, W.W., Meise, U., Gunther, V. and Kurz, M. (1994) Compliance with antipsychotic drug treatment: influence of side effects. *Acta Psychiatrica Scandinavica*, **89**, 11–15.

Fuller Torrey, E. (1994) Violent behaviour by individuals with serious mental illness. *Hospital and Community Psychiatry*, **45**, 653–662.

Gaebel, W. (1997) Towards the improvement of compliance: the significance of psychoeducation and new antipsychotic drugs. *International Clinical Psychopharmacology*, **12**(Suppl. 1), S37–S42.

Gaebel, W. and Pietzcker, A. (1985) One-year outcome of schizophrenic patients – the interaction of chronicity and neuroleptic treatment. *Pharmacopsychiatry*, **18**, 235–239.

Gottesman, I.I. (1991) *Schizophrenia Genesis. The Origins of Madness*. W.H. Freeman, New York.

Green, J.H. (1988) Frequent re-hospitalisation and non-compliance treatment. *Hospital and Community Psychiatry*, **39**, 963–966.

Guest, J.F. and Cookson, R.F. (1999) Cost of schizophrenia in the UK. *Pharmacoeconomics*, **15**, 597–610.

Hafner, H., Loffler, W., Maurer, K. *et al.* (1999) Depression, negative symptoms, social stigma and social decline in the early course of schizophrenia. Central Institute of Mental Health, Mannheim, Germany. *Acta Psychiatrica Scandinavica*, **100**, 105–118.

Haywood, T.W., Kravitz, H.M., Grossman, L.S. *et al.* (1995) Predicting the revolving door phenomenon among patients with schizophrenic, schizoaffective and affective disorders. *American Journal of Psychiatry*, **152**, 856–861.

Helgason, L. (1990) Twenty years' follow-up of first psychiatric presentation for schizophrenia: what could have been prevented? *Acta Psychiatrica Scandinavica*, **81**, 231–235.

Hillbrand, M., Spitz, R.T. and VandenBos, G.R. (1997) Investigating the role of lipids in mood, aggression and schizophrenia. *Psychiatric Services (Washington, DC)*, **48**, 875–876.

Hoge, S.K., Applebaum, P.S., Lawlor, T. *et al.* (1990) A prospective multi-centre study of patients' refusal of antipsychotic medication. *Archives of General Psychiatry*, **47**, 949–956.

Hughes, J.R., Hatsukami, D.K., Mitchell, J.E. *et al.* (1986) Prevalence of smoking among psychiatric outpatients. *American Journal of Psychiatry*, **143**, 993–997.

Hughes, I., Hill, B. and Budd, R. (1997) Compliance with antipsychotic medication: From theory to practice. *Journal of Mental Health UK*, **6**, 473–489.

Hultman, C.M., Sparen, P., Takei, N. *et al.* (1999) Prenatal and perinatal risk factors for schizophrenia, affective psychosis and reactive psychosis of early onset: case-control study. *British Medical Journal*, **318**, 421–426.

Jones, E. (1999) The phenomenology of abnormal belief: a philosophical and psychiatric enquiry. *Philosophy, Psychiatry and Psychology*, **6**, 1–16.

Jones, P., Rodgers, B., Murray, R. and Marmot, M. (1994) Child development risk factors for adult schizophrenia in the British 1946 birth cohort. *The Lancet*, **344**, 1398–1402.

Kane, J.M. (1985) Compliance issues in outpatient treatment. *Journal of Clinical Psychopharmacology*, **5**, 22S–27S.

Kelly, C. and McCreadie, R.G. (1999) Smoking habits, current symptoms and premorbid characteristics of schizophrenic patients in Nithsdale, Scotland. *American Journal of Psychiatry*, **156**, 1751–1757.

Kemp, R. and David, A. (1997) Insight and compliance. In: Compliance and the Treatment Alliance in Serious Mental Illness (ed. B. Blackwell). Harwood Academic Publishers, Amsterdam, pp. 61–68.

Kemp, R. and Lambert, T.J.C. (1995) Insight in schizophrenia and its relationship to psychopathology. *Schizophrenia Research*, **18**, 21–28.

Kemp, R., Hayward, P., Applewhite, G. *et al.* (1996) Compliance therapy in psychotic patients: a randomised controlled trial. *British Medical Journal*, **312**, 345–349.

Kemp, R., Kirov, G., Everitt, B. *et al.* (1998) Randomised controlled trial of compliance therapy. 18 month follow-up. *British Journal of Psychiatry*, **172**, 413–419.

Kissling, W. (1994) Compliance, quality assurance and standards for relapse prevention in schizophrenia. *Acta Psychiatrica Scandinavica*, **89**, 16–24.

Kissling, W., Kane, J.M., Barnes, S.J. *et al.* (1991) Guidelines for neuroleptic relapse prevention in schizophrenia: towards a consensus view. In: *Schizophrenia* (ed. W.W. Kissling). Springer, Berlin, pp. 155–163.

Kraepelin, E. (1919) Praecox and paraphrenia. E. & S. Livingstone, Edinburgh.

Ley, P. (1992) The problem of patients' non-compliance. In: *Communicating With Patients. Improving Communication, Satisfaction and Compliance.* Chapman & Hall, London.

Lieberman, J.A. (1996) Atypical antipsychotic drugs as a first-line treatment of schizophrenia: a rationale and hypothesis. *Journal of Clinical Psychiatry*, **57**(Suppl. 11), 68–71.

Lieberman, J.A. (1998) *Re-integration of the Schizophrenic Patient.* Science Press, London.

Lieberman, J., Jody, D., Geisler, S. *et al.* (1993) Time course and biologic correlates of treatment response in first-episode schizophrenia. *Archives of General Psychiatry*, **50**, 369–376.

McEvoy, J.P., Apperson, L.J., Applebaum, P.S. *et al.* (1989) Insight in schizophrenia. Its relationship to acute psychopathology. *Journal of Nervous and Mental Disease*, **177**, 43–47.

McGuffin, P., Owen, M.J., O'Donovan, M. *et al.* (1994) *Seminars in Psychiatric Genetics*. Gaskel Press, London.

Macpherson, R., Jerrom, B. and Hughes, A. (1996) A controlled study of education about drug treatment in schizophrenia. *British Journal of Psychiatry*, **168**, 709–717.

Maier, W. and Schwab, S. (1998) Molecular genetics of schizophrenia. *Current Opinion in Psychiatry*, **11**, 19–25.

Maier, W., Lichterman, D., Minges, J. *et al.* (1992) Schizoaffective disorder and affective disorders with mood-congruent psychotic features: keep separate or combine? Evidence from a family study. *American Journal of Psychiatry*, **149**, 1666–1673.

Marsh, L., Suddath, R.L., Higgins, N. *et al.* (1994) Medial temporal lobe structures in schizophrenia: relationship of size to duration of illness. *Schizophrenia Bulletin*, **11**, 225–238.

Matthysee, S. (1977) The role of dopamine in schizophrenia. In: *Neuroregulators and Psychiatric Disorders* (ed. E. Usdin, D. Hamburg and J. Barchas). Oxford University Press, New York.

Meltzer, H.Y., Bastani, B., Young Kwon, K. *et al.* (1989) A prospective study of clozapine in treatment-resistant schizophrenic patients. *Psychopharmacology*, **99**, 568–572.

Mikhail, B. (1981) The health belief model: a review and critical evaluation of the model, research and practice. *Advances in Nursing Science*, **4**, 65–80.

Munetz, M.R. and Benjamin, S. (1988) How to examine patients using the Abnormal Involuntary Movement Scale. *Hospital and Community Psychiatry*, **39**, 1772–1777.

Roberts, G.W., Leigh, P.N. and Weinberger, D.R. (1993) *Neuropsychiatric Disorders*. Wolfe Medical, London.

Sanz, M., Constable, G., Lopez-Ibor, I. *et al.* (1998) A comparative study of insight scales and their relationship to psychopathological and clinical variables. *Psychological Medicine*, **28**, 437–446.

Selemon, L.D., Rajkowska, G. and Goldman-Rakic, P.S. (1995) Abnormally high neuronal density in the schizophrenic cortex: a morphometric analysis of prefrontal area 9 and occipital area 17. *Archives of General Psychiatry*, **52**, 805–818.

Sheringham, J. (1999) Gender differences in brains of patients with schizophrenia: a volumetric MRI study. *American Journal of Psychiatry*, **156**, 603–609.

Strauss, J.S., Carpenter, W.T. and Bartko, J.J. (1974) The diagnosis and understanding of schizophrenia: part III. Speculations on the processes that underlie schizophrenic signs and symptoms. *Schizophrenia Bulletin*, **1**, 61–69.

Streicker, S.K., Amdur, M. and Dincin, J. (1986) Educating patients about psychiatric medication: failure to enhance compliance. *Psychosocial Rehabilitation Journal*, **4**, 15–28.

Verghese, A., John, J.K., Rajkumar, S. and Richard, J. (1989) Factors associated with the course and outcome of schizophrenia in India: results of a two-year multicentre follow-up study. *British Journal of Psychiatry*, **154**, 499–503.

Weinberger, D.R. (1987) Implications of normal brain development for the pathogenesis of schizophrenia. *Archives of General Psychiatry*, **44**, 660–668.

Wyatt, R.J. (1991) Neuroleptics and the natural course of schizophrenia. *Schizophrenia Bulletin*, **17**, 325–351.

Wyatt, R.J. (1995) Early intervention for schizophrenia: can the course of the illness be altered? *Biological Psychiatry*, 38, 1–3.

SELF-TEST QUESTIONS

1. What is the lifetime prevalence of schizophrenia?
   a. 1%
   b. 2%
   c. 5%
   d. 10%
2. What are the most prominent early symptoms of schizophrenia?
   a. Hallucinations and delusions
   b. Multiple personalities
   c. Inability to perform activities of daily living
   d. Confusion
3. Which of the following best describes the prodromal phase?
   a. Period of childhood
   b. Period characterised by subtle, non-specific symptoms of illness
   c. Period characterised by chaotic positive symptoms
   d. Period during which negative symptoms are prominent
4. Which of the following are examples of positive symptoms of schizophrenia?
   a. Social withdrawal and blunted affect
   b. Avolition and apathy
   c. Hallucinations and delusions
   d. Thought blocking and poverty of speech
5. Which best describes the role of genetics in the development of schizophrenia?
   a. Schizophrenia is a polygenic disorder in which the combined action of these genes produces vulnerability in the individual
   b. Schizophrenia is a single-gene disorder
   c. Genetics play no part in the development of schizophrenia
   d. None of the above
6. Which of the following have been suggested to play a role in the development of schizophrenia in some people?
   a. Perinatal hypoxia
   b. Perinatal viral infections
   c. Rhesus incompatibility
   d. All of the above
7. In which of the following pathways is a neurochemical disturbance hypothesised to produce positive symptoms of schizophrenia?
   a. Nigrostriatal dopamine pathway
   b. Tuberoinfundibular dopamine pathway
   c. Mesocortical dopamine pathway
   d. Mesolimbic dopamine pathway
8. Drug-induced neurochemical disturbance in the nigrostriatal dopamine pathway produces which of the following side-effects?
   a. Sedation

   b.   Weight gain
   c.   Extrapyramidal side-effects
   d.   Constipation

9.   Atypical antipsychotics:
   a.   Only block dopamine receptors in the mesolimbic dopamine pathway
   b.   Do not produce extrapyramidal side-effects
   c.   Do not block dopamine receptors
   d.   Are more effective than conventional antipsychotics in the treatment of positive symptoms

10.   Prolonged blockade of dopamine receptors in the nigrostriatal dopamine pathway, leading to their upregulation, may produce a condition known as:
   a.   Neuroleptic malignant syndrome
   b.   Tardive dyskinesia
   c.   Parkinsonism
   d.   Amenorrhoea

11.   Which of the following atypical antipsychotics is licensed for treatment-resistant schizophrenia?
   a.   Olanzapine
   b.   Risperidone
   c.   Quetiapine
   d.   Clozapine

12.   Clozapine is a drug that is metabolised by some of the cytochrome P450 enzymes. The clinical consequence of this is that:
   a.   Smokers may need higher doses of clozapine than non-smokers
   b.   The dose of clozapine may need to be lowered when given concomitantly with an SSRI
   c.   The dose of clozapine may need to be reduced when taken concomitantly with the antibiotic erythromycin
   d.   All of the above

13.   Adherence to treatment is improved by:
   a.   Acceptance of illness
   b.   Perception of susceptibility
   c.   Positive therapeutic alliance
   d.   All of the above

DEMENTIA

6

INTRODUCTION

Dementia, literally meaning 'out of mind', is classified as a syndrome caused by disease of the brain. It is acquired and is chronic or progressive in nature, thus distinguishing it from learning disabilities and acute organic brain syndromes, and is usually irreversible. It is characterised by disturbances in higher cortical functions such as memory, thinking, orientation, comprehension and language. There is no clouding of consciousness (Lishman 1987). These cognitive symptoms are often accompanied by psychiatric symptoms such as hallucinations and delusions and there is an associated social decline and loss of independence. The International Classification of Diseases (ICD-10) refers to dementia as a syndrome 'due to disease of the brain, usually of a chronic or progressive nature, in which there is disturbance of multiple higher cortical functions, including memory, thinking, orientation, comprehension, calculation, learning capacity, language and judgement'. Most definitions of dementia refer to the global nature of the impairments: the incapacity associated with dementia is more extensive than can be accounted for by focal brain damage. Dementia occurs in Alzheimer's disease, in cerebrovascular disease and in other conditions that affect the brain.

> Dementia is a syndrome due to disease of the brain, usually of a chronic or progressive nature, in which there is disturbance of multiple higher cortical functions, including memory, thinking, orientation, comprehension, calculation, learning capacity, language and judgement.

◀ **Key point**

Dementia produces a significant decline in intellectual functioning and compromises the individual's ability to carry out personal activities of daily living such as washing, dressing and eating. This decline forms the primary requirement for a diagnosis of dementia. The most common cognitive deficits experienced by someone with dementia can be grouped under the following headings:

- amnesia (impairment of memory)
- aphasia (difficulties in communicating)
- apraxia (loss of the ability to perform previously learned motor tasks)
- agnosia (inability to recognise previously learned sensory input).

> The most common cognitive deficits experienced by someone with dementia are amnesia, aphasia, apraxia and agnosia.

◀ **Key point**

The most common symptom of dementia is difficulty in remembering things. We have two types of memory, short-term and long-term. Our short-term memory is responsible for us remembering things that happened only a short time ago, whereas our long-term memory enables us to remember things that happened in the distant past. The hippocampus processes short-term memories while long-term memories are stored in the cortex. The hippocampus begins losing neurones in significant numbers from middle age and is severely affected in many dementias. The consequence for the individual is impaired short-term memory. Long-term memory, however, by virtue of it being stored in the cortex, remains intact until much later in the disease.

However, complaints of memory impairment in older people are common. Could it be, therefore, that dementia is an inevitable consequence of ageing for all of us should we live long enough? Age-associated memory impairments, probably caused by neurochemical changes in the brain related to ageing, do not produce the progressive decline associated with dementia. The consensus of opinion is that dementia is more than simple ageing, although the longer we live the greater the likelihood of us developing dementia.

Key point ▶

> Age-associated memory impairments, probably caused by neurochemical changes in the brain related to ageing, do not produce the progressive decline associated with dementia.

Dementia has become one of the most challenging medical problems of the 21st century. Its prevalence rises with age, with 6% of the population over 65 being affected (Kay *et al.*, 1970). This rises rapidly the older we get, reaching a prevalence of around 40% by the age of 95. The Alzheimer's Research Trust estimates that there are 800 000 sufferers of dementia in the UK. The commonest cause of dementia is Alzheimer's disease, responsible for about two-thirds of all cases. The remainder is made up mostly of vascular dementia and Lewy body dementia. Some dementias result from a treatable cause and can therefore be reversed if treated early. Classification of the dementias has become more sophisticated, with different subtypes being identified according to clinical presentation and representing different underlying pathological processes.

Memory, particularly short-term memory, is often the first area of functioning to be affected in an individual. Other areas of intellectual impairment follow, such as the loss of the ability for abstract reasoning, and disorientation. Thought disorder may be present and affective symptoms often accompany the early stages. It can be difficult to distinguish between a major affective disorder and dementia. A diagnosis of dementia is achieved through a full mental status and neurological evaluation. Identifying dementia in its early stages can be difficult. Carers will often cover up any deficits experienced by their loved one and it is often the sudden loss of support, perhaps through the death of a spouse, that leads to a crisis. By this stage the dementia is often well established.

Behavioural patterns change in early dementia. For example, when attempting to answer questions, patients will often give irrelevant answers, make gestures indicating that the answer is on the tip of their tongue, or smile and give no response at all. They may take offence at the questions and become tearful or aggressive. There is also a tendency towards preoccupation with diaries and calendars, loss of interest in hobbies and exaggerated satisfaction with the completion of trivial tasks. The early identification of dementia clearly benefits from the observations of someone who knows the patient well.

> The commonest cause of dementia is Alzheimer's disease, accounting for about two-thirds of all cases.

◀ **Key point**

ALZHEIMER'S DISEASE

Clinical picture

Alzheimer's disease is a degenerative disease of the brain with characteristic neuropathological and neurochemical features. Its onset is usually insidious and the disease develops over several years, the prevalence doubling with every 5 years over the age of 65. The number of cases of Alzheimer's disease worldwide is estimated to be 12 million (Alzheimer's Disease International, 2002). It is expected that the numbers will rise to 36 million cases in the developed world by 2050 (Katzman, 2000). Alzheimer's disease affects more than 10% of people over the age of 65 living in the community and more than half of those living in nursing homes. It lags behind only heart disease, cancer and stroke as the leading cause of death in industrialised nations and as such represents a major burden on the economy. Onset of the disease is typically late in life, although Alzheimer's disease of presenile onset (i.e. with onset before the age of 65) also occurs. In this type there is often a family history of a similar dementia. Alzheimer's disease is more common in women than in men.

> Alzheimer's disease affects over 10% of people over the age of 65 living in the community, and more than half of those living in nursing homes.

◀ **Key point**

A diagnosis of dementia is based on clinical features meeting the diagnostic criteria of ICD-10. Alzheimer's disease, by definition, is a disease with certain pathological features and a definitive diagnosis can therefore only be made *post-mortem*. However, a probable diagnosis of Alzheimer's disease is made based on the presenting clinical features of the dementia, primarily impairment of memory, thinking, judgement

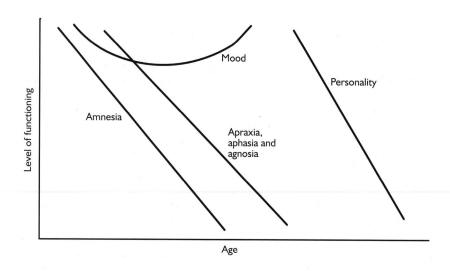

Figure 6.1

Variable progression of symptoms in Alzheimer's disease

and higher cortical functioning, as well as other features such as disordered behaviour. The disparity between individuals with regard to their clinical symptomatology is the result of random damage to the brain caused by the degenerative process. Hence, no two individuals present with the same clinical picture, since no two patterns of brain damage are the same. The challenge to the health-care professional is therefore great and made all the more difficult by the variable progression of the disease (Figure 6.1).

The progression of Alzheimer's disease tends to be slow for the first 5–10 years, amnesia being the prominent early sign of its existence. Kopelman (1985) studied memory in people with Alzheimer's disease and concluded that they had defects in both memory capacity and retention and memory acquisition. He interpreted the anterograde memory problems faced by these individuals, in which there is impaired recall and recognition of postmorbid experiences, as a consequence of the inability to take in new information. No explanation is given for the retrograde amnesia also suffered by these patients, in which there is impaired recall and recognition of premorbid experiences.

Impaired short-term memory is the major symptom of the early stages of Alzheimer's disease, although long-term memory tends to remain intact until much later in the disease. This provides a challenge for the clinician, who must be able to recognise the disparity for what it is and not misinterpret a lack of short-term memory as being difficult behaviour simply because the patient is able to recall memories from their past. Many patients will try and compensate for their poor short-term memory by using memory cues such as notes, or rely more heavily on their long-term memory. We often hear it said that our patients are living in the past!

Key point ▶

> People with Alzheimer's disease have defects in both memory capacity and retention and memory acquisition.

Patients with Alzheimer's disease also commonly experience aphasia – difficulty in communicating. It is useful to think of aphasia in terms of receptive aphasia and expressive aphasia. **Receptive aphasia**, found in the middle to late stages of Alzheimer's disease, is essentially a problem of recognising language. The patient is able to receive sound in the normal way but selective damage to the auditory association cortex, caused by the disease, renders the patient unable to make sense of the sounds (Benson 1994). Practitioners must be aware that what they say to patients is often not understood and that the actions that follow can be seen as threatening in the absence of understanding. This can lead to confrontation and the patient becomes labelled as difficult. Imagine being asked to come to the dining room for dinner and not understanding this request. When the practitioner later returns to find you have not gone to the dining room they immediately take you by the arm and lead you there. If you have no understanding of where you are going or why, you are likely to feel threatened and may react by resisting the attempts of the practitioner. A common scenario is that the patient is thought of as being difficult to manage and is given antipsychotic medication. This will have no beneficial effects and is likely to lead to other problems for the patient. Skilful communicators are essential if these problems are to be avoided.

Expressive aphasia is impaired use of language skills, including difficulty in constructing sentences, finding words and naming objects. Damage to the motor language area in the brain known as Broca's area produces the difficulty and is common in Alzheimer's disease. Benson (1994) demonstrated that the expression of language has two components, each being produced in opposite sides of the brain. The left side of our brain is where our thoughtful speech is produced, whereas the right side is responsible for emotive language and singing. The degenerative processes occurring in Alzheimer's disease are not uniform and it is often the case that the motor language area in the left-brain is selectively damaged. This leads to expressive aphasia and the patient is unable to get their message across. The ability to sing or speak when emotionally charged remains intact. How often do we see patients unable to put simple sentences together, like a request to go to the toilet, and able to sing an entire song or swear profusely when angry or threatened? It is important that practitioners and carers alike recognise the nature of expressive aphasia and do not fall into the trap of thinking that their patient/relative should be able to express themselves, simply because they can sing a song.

Patients with Alzheimer's disease commonly experience aphasia, difficulty in communicating.

◀ *Key point*

We are not born with the ability to be able to feed ourselves, dress ourselves or even walk. We learn these complex motor tasks over many years, only later to take them for granted. Benson (1994) describes the cognitive deficit experienced by people with Alzheimer's disease, apraxia, as the inability to perform previously learned motor tasks. Apraxias fall into the three main categories of feeding apraxia, activities of daily living apraxia and gait apraxia. The level of degeneration leading to impairment in any one area seems to be random, resulting in patients losing the ability to perform some quite simple tasks while retaining abilities in other more complex areas.

Key point ▶

> Apraxia is the inability to perform previously learned motor tasks. Apraxias associated with Alzheimer's disease include feeding apraxia, activities of daily living apraxia and gait apraxia

Feeding apraxia is the loss of the skills required for feeding oneself in a socially acceptable way. During childhood we learn how to behave during a meal, ranging from the use of cutlery to general table manners. People with Alzheimer's disease lose these abilities and revert back to the level of skill they had in their childhood. How often do we see patients eating food with their fingers when a knife and fork would be more appropriate, or taking food from each other? Relearning these skills is not a feasible option in Alzheimer's disease. We generally work with the impairment by providing practical aids such as easy-to-hold cutlery and non-slip mats for the plates, and provide foods that can be eaten easily with the fingers if appropriate.

Another dimension to feeding apraxia is the reduced ability of the patient to chew and swallow food. Special diets can be provided to address this difficulty. Feeding apraxia, as with many other aspects of Alzheimer's disease, tends to worsen as the disease progresses.

Activities of daily living apraxias include such things as the inability to wash and dress and attend to toilet needs. Practitioners need to be sensitive to individual needs and a great deal of support may be required. Because of the discrete nature of the damage to the brain, the care given must be tailored to that individual. One patient may retain skills lost by another and it is important that the patient is allowed to continue to use the skills they have. If they do not, they risk losing them, making them ever more dependent.

We take the ability to walk for granted and yet it is easy to see the profound effects brain injury, such as that sustained in a stroke, has on our gait. It should not be surprising, therefore, that the dementia associated with Alzheimer's disease produces **gait apraxia**, or inability to walk, in its later stages. Benson (1994) describes severe damage of the prefrontal and parietal cortices in Alzheimer's disease as the major factor in gait apraxia. Other areas of the brain responsible for less intricate movement of the limbs tend to remain intact longer, allowing patients to retain the ability to get out of bed, for instance. The implications are obvious – patients will often have their movement restricted to avoid the probable injury that would result from a fall.

The final common cognitive deficit experienced by patients who have

Alzheimer's disease is **agnosia**, described by Benson (1994) as the inability to recognise previously learned sensory input. In much the same way as receptive aphasia restricts a hearing patient from understanding what is being said to them, visual agnosia restricts a patient with good eyesight from recognising what is before them, such as family and friends. Damage to the visual association cortex is the problem here and may even result in the individual not recognising his/her own reflection. This can be very distressing and may warrant the removal of mirrors from that person's environment. Agnosia can also be extended to other senses, such as olfactory and visceral information. A gas leak may not be recognised for what it is or the individual may not recognise the need to go to the toilet when the bladder is distended.

Agnosia, the inability to recognise previously learned sensory input, is a common cognitive deficit experienced by patients who have Alzheimer's disease.

◀ *Key point*

Alzheimer's disease progresses through three phases. The first or early stage is characterised by amnesia and subtle apraxia, particularly in the activities of daily living. There may be some early aphasia and the individual often experiences anxiety and depression in response to this decline. As the disease progresses through the middle phase there is a worsening of the amnesia and gradual loss of independence in activities of daily living. The need for supervision increases and there is often a disruption of the normal sleep–wake cycle. The vocabulary of the person becomes very limited as the late phase nears. The late phase is marked by a total breakdown of personality and intellectual function.

CASE STUDY 6.1   MARY, A CLIENT WITH ALZHEIMER'S DISEASE

Read this case study and then attempt to answer the questions that follow.

Mary is a 74-year-old woman who has recently been widowed. She lives alone, although her daughter lives nearby. Since the death of her husband, concerns have grown that Mary is finding it difficult to cope. She has experienced progressive memory loss for the past 3-4 years, which has become more apparent now that she is living independently. For instance, Mary often forgets to lock the door when she goes out.

Mary, previously a very house-proud lady, has allowed her house to become dirty and littered with hazards. She is also neglecting her personal hygiene and the house has a distinct smell of urine. Mary has had several mishaps in the kitchen, including setting fire to pans and boiling an empty kettle. Mary's daughter is becoming very concerned about her mother's safety and has tried to offer more assistance in the home. This offer has been rebuffed, Mary seemingly not understanding the nature of the offer and often not recognising her daughter when she sees her. This situation has escalated to the degree that Mary now locks herself in the house and is abusive towards her daughter. She believes her daughter is an intruder who is trying to steal her money.

Consider Mary's case and identify the nature of the difficulties she is experiencing. Categorise these under the headings amnesia, aphasia, apraxia and agnosia.

Severe motor defects are apparent and the individual is often incontinent. The progression towards death is variable and unpredictable.

Aetiology

The German neurologist Alois Alzheimer first reported the signs and symptoms and *post-mortem* brain pathology that define Alzheimer's disease. The pathological changes associated with Alzheimer's disease can be described in terms of both macroscopic and microscopic alterations. Macroscopic changes can include cortical atrophy, producing marked reduction in the gyri (the folded outer surfaces of the brain) and widening of the sulci (the ridges of the brain that separate the gyri). There is also likely to be dilation of the ventricles, the cerebrospinal-fluid-filled cavities of the brain.

Modern brain imaging techniques such as magnetic resonance imaging (MRI) and computed tomography (CT) scans provide clinicians with sophisticated images detailing the extent of cerebral atrophy. Charting the progression of Alzheimer's disease has been achieved using positron emission tomography (PET). The results of these investigations have provided evidence that Alzheimer's disease is different from normal ageing and that it is not a diffuse disease. They also suggest that presenile and senile dementia are the same. The future use of imaging techniques may allow for more sophisticated prescribing of treatments, including better differentiation of dementia and depression.

Microscopic changes associated with Alzheimer's disease are quite variable but distinct from ageing. The presence of neuritic plaques with amyloid cores and neurofibrillary tangles of abnormally phosphorylated tau proteins are the defining features. Neuritic plaques are extracellular lesions with beta-amyloid deposits, formed from the abnormal processes of neurones, possibly axons or dendrites. Their significance is unclear and opinion is divided as to whether they are degenerative or regenerative structures. What is clear is that these plaques can be found in small numbers in the brains of people who do not have Alzheimer's disease and are presumed to be a consequence of ageing. For a diagnosis of Alzheimer's disease, the number of plaques is of greater significance than their mere presence.

The second major pathological change associated with Alzheimer's disease is the formation of neurofibrillary tangles, intracellular disruption of the neurone's microtubules. It is hypothesised that tau proteins become abnormally phosphorylated, leading to the twisting together of microtubules and consequent death of the neurone. Unlike neuritic plaques, the presence of neurofibrillary tangles as a consequence of ageing is unlikely and is far more likely to be indicative of a neurodegenerative disease.

Key point ▶

> Microscopic changes associated with Alzheimer's disease include the presence of neuritic plaques with amyloid cores and neurofibrillary tangles of abnormally phosphorylated tau proteins.

Autosomal dominant inheritance has been mooted for Alzheimer's disease, the existence of identical twins with the disorder providing some evidence for this (Kilpatrick *et al.*, 1983). The case for Alzheimer's disease being inherited is strongest when its onset is in the presenile period. The more common late-onset Alzheimer's disease does not show the clear clustering in families seen with the early-onset form. It is, however, generally considered to be the product of the interaction between genetic and environmental factors. Recent studies into the presence of susceptibility genes for late-onset Alzheimer's disease have been summarised by Craddock and Lendon (1998).

> The evidence for autosomal dominant inheritance of Alzheimer's disease is strongest when its onset is in the presenile period.

◀ **Key point**

The possibility of genes being responsible for the pathological changes associated with Alzheimer's disease has led to the search for predictive tests for both early- and late-onset disease. However, the present lack of effective treatment means that genetic screening is of little value and should only be used in families known to be at high risk and then only in conjunction with genetic counselling.

Three genes have been identified as possible candidates for the development of Alzheimer's disease. The first gene, found on chromosome 21, is linked to the synthesis of amyloid precursor protein (APP). The amyloid cascade hypothesis is one of the contemporary theories for the biological basis of Alzheimer's disease. The second gene, thought to be responsible for more cases of Alzheimer's disease than that found on chromosome 21, is linked to the presence of amyloid plaques and is found on chromosome 14. Finally, a gene found on chromosome 19 responsible for the synthesis of apolipoprotein E (Apo-E), is associated with late-onset Alzheimer's disease. Apo-E is found in both plaques and tangles and is thought to stabilise tau protein, a protein associated with the formation of the microtubules essential for the transport of materials from the nucleus to the dendrites of the cell.

> Three genes, found on chromosome 21, 14 and 19, have been identified as possible candidates for the development of Alzheimer's disease.

◀ **Key point**

Amyloid cascade hypothesis

The amyloid cascade hypothesis of Alzheimer's disease theorises that the disease is caused by the excessive presence of beta-amyloid, leading to the destruction of neurones. It is unclear as to whether this excess is due to overproduction or under-removal of the protein. The production of APP may be compromised by a genetic abnormality that leads to the formation of beta-amyloid deposits and ultimately plaques and tangles. Alternatively, there may be a problem with Apo-E, the protein responsible for the removal of beta-amyloid. If the Apo-E is unable to properly bind with and remove beta-amyloid, the resulting build-up of amyloid destroys neurones and goes on to produce the symptoms of Alzheimer's disease. Future treatments for Alzheimer's disease aim to halt the progression of the disease by altering the synthesis of either APP or Apo-E.

Key point ▶

> The amyloid cascade hypothesis of Alzheimer's disease theorises that the disease is caused by the excessive presence of beta-amyloid, leading to the destruction of neurones.

Cholinergic hypothesis

The cholinergic system is believed to play a role in many of the behaviours associated with Alzheimer's disease, particularly those of attention and memory. This is evidenced by a positive correlation between cholinergic neurone loss and degree of dementia. A leading theory for the symptom of amnesia in Alzheimer's disease is based on the idea that a loss of cholinergic functioning due to the deposition of beta-amyloid in these neurones leads to the disruption of memory, whether this be the result of ageing or the pathological changes associated with Alzheimer's disease.

Key point ▶

> A loss of cholinergic functioning due to the deposition of beta-amyloid in cholinergic neurones may be responsible for the amnesia associated with Alzheimer's disease.

Many of the cholinergic neurones believed to be responsible for short-term memory have their cell bodies in the nucleus basalis of Meynert, an area of the basal forebrain. It is possible that degeneration of the nucleus basalis is responsible for the short-term memory problems seen in normal ageing. It is also possible that the degeneration of cholinergic neurones seen in Alzheimer's disease starts in the nucleus basalis and progresses to the profound memory disturbance character-istic of the disease. Procholinergic agents, which enhance the production of acetylcholine, have been shown to improve memory in people with Alzheimer's disease, although these improvements are generally limited and mostly transient.

Excitotoxic hypothesis

Excitotoxicity is a process whereby neurones degenerate as a conse-quence of excessive neurotransmission in the excitatory glutamate neurones. It has been implicated in a variety of neurodegenerative disorders such as Alzheimer's disease, Parkinson's disease and stroke. Excitotoxicity may also be involved in psychosis, mania and other symptoms of mental illness. The excitotoxicity occurring here may be a normal process that is out of control. This gives some explanation for the observation that late treatment of psychosis reduces the likelihood of the individual responding to treatment when it is eventually commenced. This forms the basis of the argument for early pharmacological intervention in psychosis.

Excitotoxicity, a process whereby neurones degenerate as a consequence of excessive neurotransmission in the excitatory glutamate neurones, has been implicated in Alzheimer's disease.

◀ **Key point**

It is believed that neurodegeneration occurs through excitotoxicity produced at the *N*-methyl-D-aspartate (NMDA) glutamate receptor. This receptor is part of a complex that controls the movement of calcium into the neurone. Opening of the channel produces greater excitation of the neurone. The excitotoxicity produced by the excessive opening of the ion channel may be slow, as in disorders such as Alzheimer's disease, or very fast, as may be the case with stroke.

Cell-cycle hypothesis

Researchers have discovered that the death of neurones in Alzheimer's disease is preceded by a failed attempt at cell division. In other words, Alzheimer's disease is a disease of cell-cycle dysfunction (Habeck 2001). Could Alzheimer's disease be regarded as a form of cancer? This analogy might not be relevant, as neurones in the adult brain are unable to divide. However, this hypothesis may potentially lead to new strategies for the treatment of Alzheimer's disease.

PHARMACOLOGICAL TREATMENT

Before considering the pharmacological treatment of Alzheimer's disease it is worth thinking about the implications of using medications in older people in general. Ageing increases the sensitivity of individuals to medications as a result of pharmacodynamic and pharmacokinetic changes. Reduced numbers of neurones and receptors, alongside altered absorption, distribution, metabolism and excretion of drugs, produce this increased sensitivity and necessitate vigilance in ensuring that the lowest effective dosage of medication is used. Polypharmacy – the use of combinations of medications – should be avoided, since the elderly are at increased risk of complications caused by drug interactions. Drugs should also be given longer to work. For example, Georgotas *et al.* (1989) showed that antidepressants might take as long as 8 weeks to provide any benefit in the elderly. It is also important to avoid the use of drugs that are likely to increase the risk of falls, especially the sedative-hypnotics. The elderly are particularly sensitive to orthostatic hypotension. Finally, drugs with a high degree of anticholinergic activity should be avoided.

Key point ▶

> Polypharmacy should be avoided wherever possible in the elderly as they are at increased risk of complications caused by drug interactions.

In July 2000 the Alzheimer's Society submitted an appraisal of the drugs for Alzheimer's disease to the UK National Institute for Clinical Excellence. In this appraisal concern was expressed about the excessive and inappropriate use of neuroleptic medication in people with Alzheimer's disease. Neuroleptics can often be inappropriately prescribed for the management of challenging behaviour, including aggression and wandering. The appraisal recommended a more client-centred approach to the pharmacological treatment of people with dementia. The appraisal also recommends a more widespread use of the acetylcholinesterase treatments. While not offering a cure, these drugs may be valuable in delaying the onset of the symptoms of Alzheimer's disease and in restoring skills deficits for a period of time. The *National Service Framework for Older People* (Department of Health, 2001) also makes reference to medicines and older people, stating that older people should gain the maximum benefit from their medication to maintain or increase their quality and duration of life but should not suffer unnecessarily from illness caused by excessive, inappropriate or inadequate consumption of medicines.

Key point ▶

> Older people should gain the maximum benefit from their medication to maintain or increase their quality and duration of life but not suffer unnecessarily from illness caused by excessive, inappropriate or inadequate consumption of medicines.

Some of the early forms of pharmacological treatment for Alzheimer's disease focused on the use of precursors for acetylcholine synthesis. These proved unsuccessful in clinical trials and have been superseded by treatments that aim to increase the levels of acetylcholine by other mechanisms. The pharmacological agents **donepezil hydrochloride, rivastigmine** and **galantamine** have produced good results and work by blocking acetylcholinesterase, the enzyme responsible for the breakdown of acetylcholine. The consequence of this inhibition is a build up in the levels of acetylcholine to such an extent that cholinergic activity is significantly enhanced. The need for the presence of functioning cholinergic neurones has restricted the use of such agents for mild to moderate Alzheimer's disease.

There is no evidence that these drugs arrest the progressive degeneration of neurones characteristic of the disease and they therefore do not improve the long-term prognosis for an individual. (There is some evidence that acetylcholinesterase inhibitors may slow the course of the underlying degenerative process in some patients.) There is, however, substantial evidence supporting the use of acetylcholinesterase inhibitors to enhance memory and general quality of life in the short term for individuals in the early stages of the disease. Users of these drugs and their carers highlight three main areas of improvement associated with the taking of the drug. These are improvement in mood, reduction in fear and distress and improvement in confidence.

> Acetylcholinesterase inhibitors aim to increase the levels of acetylcholine by blocking acetylcholinesterase, the enzyme responsible for the breakdown of acetylcholine.

◀ **Key point**

The difficulty in making an early diagnosis of Alzheimer's disease, when the use of acetylcholinesterase inhibitors would be most beneficial, is a problem. Variable response also makes the use of these agents problematic. Individuals who respond best can show considerable improvement, which is noticeable to both the patient and his/her carer (Figure 6.2). This improvement may be noticeable after just a few weeks and be sustained for many months. It is more common, however, for the improvement to be noticeable only to the practitioner and their carer, rather than the patient him/herself. The improvement typically lasts around 6 months, after which time the decline has reached pretreatment levels (Figure 6.2). Withdrawal of the treatment results in a steady decline to a level of functioning that would have been expected had treatment never commenced. There are still others for whom the initiation of acetylcholinesterase inhibitors produces no improvement but does slow the expected rate of decline (Figure 6.2). It is unlikely that the initiation of treatment will worsen a patient's condition.

The need for regular reviews of the prescribing of the acetylcholinesterase inhibitors is essential. Counselling explaining the nature of the treatment and the benefits and risks associated with its use, including the likelihood of treatment failure, should always support the

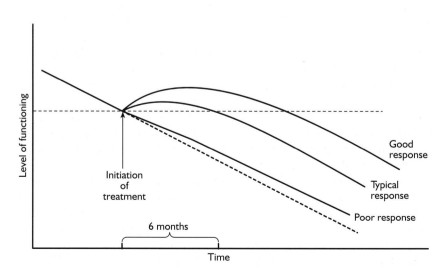

Figure 6.2

Variable response to treatment with acetylcholinesterase inhibitors prescribing of acetylcholinesterase inhibitors. The person taking the drug must be able to consent to its use.

Counselling explaining the nature of the treatment and the benefits and risks associated with their use, including the likelihood of treatment failure, should always support the prescribing of acetylcholinesterase inhibitors.

Taylor *et al.* (2001) recommend a generic protocol for the drug treatment of Alzheimer's disease. The use of acetylcholinesterase inhibitors is based on cognitive tests, such as the Mini Mental State Examination (MMSE). Evidence suggests that acetylcholinesterase inhibitors are only effective in patients with mild to moderate illness, those having a MMSE score of 10–24. If the drug is tolerated (adverse effects include nausea, vomiting and diarrhoea) further cognitive tests are performed at regular predetermined intervals to assess whether the patient is showing signs of improvement. A change of 3 points on the MMSE score is considered by some to be a measure of improvement, although others consider that a failure to deteriorate over 3–6 months is a measure of response when set against an expected cognitive decline in untreated Alzheimer's disease over this period.

Patients who do not meet the criteria for improvement should have the treatment withdrawn and be given supportive counselling. Inevitably all patients receiving acetylcholinesterase inhibitors will have their treatment withdrawn at some point. It is worth remembering that all drugs with anticholinergic effects will reduce the efficacy of the acetylcholinesterase inhibitors and should therefore be avoided.

Key point ▶

Evidence suggests that acetylcholinesterase inhibitors are only effective in patients with mild to moderate illness, those having a MMSE score of 10–24.

The acetylcholinesterase inhibitors have been systematically reviewed to assess their clinical efficacy and safety for patients with Alzheimer's disease. These reviews are available in the Cochrane Library. Donepezil was reviewed in patients with mild to moderate Alzheimer's disease treated for periods of 12, 24 or 52 weeks. Modest improvements were produced in cognitive function and global clinical state, although patient self-assessment of quality of life showed no improvement (Birks *et al.*, 2002a). Rivastigmine also showed benefits for people with mild to moderate Alzheimer's disease, particularly in the areas of cognitive function, activities of daily living and severity of dementia (Birks *et al.*, 2002b). Similar results were found for galantamine when used with mild to moderately impaired patients (Olin and Schneider 2002).

The use of acetylcholinesterase inhibitors is currently limited to the treatment of memory disturbance in Alzheimer's disease. As our understanding increases of the role that cholinergic neurones play in Alzheimer's disease, it is likely that the use of acetylcholinesterase inhibitors will extend in the future to include the treatment of the behavioural problems associated with the disease. Evidence is already mounting for the synergistic effects of these agents with atypical antipsychotics in the management of behavioural problems. Acetylcholinesterase inhibitors may even find a role in the treatment of disorders such as attention deficit disorder and bipolar disorder.

◄ *Key point*

It is likely that the use of acetylcholinesterase inhibitors will grow in the future to include the treatment of the behavioural problems associated with Alzheimer's disease.

As previously stated, Alzheimer's disease is more common in women than in men. As many as three times more women have Alzheimer's disease than men. While women tend to live longer than men and are therefore at greater risk of developing the disease, this cannot wholly account for the difference. Where women take oestrogen replacement therapy their risk of developing Alzheimer's disease is reduced, suggesting that a postmenopausal reduction in oestrogen is a risk factor for the disease. It is hypothesised that oestrogen acts on cholinergic neurones in a way that protects against the onset of Alzheimer's disease.

◄ *Key point*

Oestrogen replacement therapy reduces the risk of women developing Alzheimer's disease.

Another interesting concept for the treatment of Alzheimer's disease is based on findings that the incidence is lower among smokers. This has led to claims that smoking has a protective effect against Alzheimer's disease. Nicotine is a cholinergic agonist that also boosts the release of acetylcholine through its presynaptic effect. However, a recent Cochrane Review (Lopez-Arrieta *et al.*, 2002) was unable to provide any evidence that nicotine is a useful treatment for Alzheimer's disease. Smoking is also a risk factor for stroke and possibly for vascular dementia. Despite these findings, the search is on for cholinergic agonists that act at both muscarinic and nicotinic cholinergic receptors as possible future treatments for Alzheimer's disease.

The NMDA-glutamate–calcium-channel complex can be allosterically modulated (i.e. its shape can be modified) by a variety of substances. The development of neuroprotective agents that could allosterically modulate the ion channel in such a way as to reduce the influx of calcium into the neurone is a current area of research into the treatment of a whole range of neurodegenerative disorders. Alternatively, neuroprotective agents may focus on the removal of the free radicals produced in the neurone by the excessive influx of calcium. Free radicals are chemicals that are destructive to cells. Vitamin E is a dietary compound that functions as an antioxidant free radical scavenger. It is currently being tested in several neurodegenerative disorders for its ability to remove harmful free radicals. A Cochrane Review (Tabet *et al.*, 2002) found insufficient evidence of efficacy of vitamin E in the treatment of people with Alzheimer's disease, although it did recommend further studies.

The lack of effective treatments for Alzheimer's disease necessitates the continued reliance on treatments for the psychiatric symptoms of the disease, such as disturbed behaviour and altered mood. Hence, antipsychotics and antidepressants are the mainstay of pharmacological treatment. However, the pharmacokinetic changes associated with ageing should always be considered when using such medications. The elderly are more sensitive to the extrapyramidal effects, orthostatic hypotension and anticholinergic effects of antipsychotics. Sedating patients may make their management easier but will increase risks in other areas, for example the risk of falls (Ray, 1992). Falls are the major cause of accidental injury in the elderly. The consequence of falls in elderly females is made worse by the presence of osteoporosis.

Sedating drugs will also exacerbate the impaired visuospatial coordination experienced by patients with dementia. Many antipsychotics have significant anticholinergic effects that have the potential for increasing the cognitive decline associated with dementia, with obvious consequences for continuing care. Antipsychotics, when they are used, should be given in much lower doses and titrated much more slowly than in younger adults. This will reduce the incidence of side-effects and increase the likelihood of gaining a therapeutic response at a lower dose. **Olanzapine**, **risperidone** and **sulpiride** are the drugs of choice (Taylor *et al.*, 2001).

Generally, drugs should be avoided, wherever possible, in the management of agitation in dementia. Agitation includes wandering, crying out and assaultive behaviour and occurs in up to 70% of patients with dementia. A Cochrane Review, conducted by Kirchner *et al.* (2002), concluded that there is no evidence to support the use of **thioridazine** in dementia and that its use may expose patients to excess side-effects. Thioridazine has particularly dangerous cardiac effects. A similar review by Lonergan *et al.* (2002) found no evidence for the use of **haloperidol** for agitation in dementia. Reassurance and direction should be given when inappropriate behaviours occur. **Moclobemide** and the selective serotonin reuptake inhibitors (SSRIs) are recommended for depressed mood.

Key point ▶

> The lack of effective treatments for Alzheimer's disease necessitates the continued reliance on treatments for the psychiatric symptoms of the disease, such as disturbed behaviour and altered mood.

While the development of treatments for Alzheimer's disease focuses on a single mechanism of action, the disease is almost certainly due to a combination of factors, all of which require treatment. Modern approaches to treatment increasingly use combinations of pharmacological agents to address the memory and cognitive disturbances alongside treatments for psychosis and disturbed mood and behaviour.

Future treatments

Alzheimer's disease results in a progressive loss of neurones. A future treatment may involve the use of growth factors to stimulate the regeneration of neurones. This approach to treatment of Alzheimer's disease is still in the preclinical phase of development. Alternatively, there may be scope for the development of neuronal transplantation techniques.

Schenk (1999) and his colleagues are currently looking at the possibility of using a vaccine in the fight against Alzheimer's disease. The vaccine aims to reduce the build up of beta-amyloid, one of the waste proteins associated with the disease. Research using mice bred with the gene responsible for the formation of amyloid plaques in humans has shown that the vaccine, made up of a small amount of insoluble beta-amyloid, stimulates an immune response in the mice that prevents the excessive build up of beta-amyloid. The mice receiving the vaccine showed a much-reduced propensity to develop the neuritic plaques indicative of Alzheimer's pathology compared with mice injected with a placebo. The vaccine was also shown to reduce neuritic plaques already formed in adult mice, raising the possibility of a vaccine that could cure symptomatic patients.

The work of Schenk (1999) is based on the theory that Alzheimer's disease is caused by the formation of neuritic plaques, rather than the plaques simply being a byproduct of the disease. Clinical trials in humans might prove unsuccessful if the mere removal of the plaques does not alter the symptoms of Alzheimer's disease. The vaccine does not take account of the formation of neurofibrillary tangles, which may prove to have greater significance in the pathology of the disease.

Another target for therapy is the enzymes involved in cholesterol homeostasis. Research has shown that altering cholesterol can influence beta-amyloid metabolism in experimental model systems and that cholesterol-lowering agents could reduce the incidence of Alzheimer's disease (Golde and Eckman 2001). The researchers believe that cholesterol influences beta-amyloid metabolism in several ways, including modification of its production, deposition and clearance. Thus, pharmacological modulation of cholesterol levels could provide a relatively safe means to reduce beta-amyloid accumulation in the brain and thereby prevent or slow the development of Alzheimer's disease.

Clinical studies in Australia and the USA are investigating approaches to prevent the deposition of beta-amyloid and dissolve the amyloid plaques associated with Alzheimer's disease (Dorrell 2001). Scientists believe the damage seen in the condition is potentiated by a build-up of metal ions, particularly copper. Clinical trials using targeted delivery of chelating agents aim to reduce beta-amyloid levels and thereby improve the symptoms of the disease.

Colostrinin, a new drug derived from mammals' first milk, is undergoing trials as a treatment for Alzheimer's disease (Owens 2001). It may stabilise Alzheimer's disease by several mechanisms, including the inhibition of amyloid plaque formation, scavenging free radicals and increasing the adhesiveness of cells in the brain.

Alzheimer's disease sufferers are known to be deficient in the enzyme responsible for converting choline into acetylcholine. It is hypothesised that extra consumption of choline may reduce the progression of dementia. Lecithin is a major dietary source of choline, although randomised trials have thus far not supported its use in dementia (Higgins and Flicker 2002).

Ginkgo biloba leaf extracts may have some efficacy in treating memory problems and dementia. A meta-analysis by Oken *et al.* (1998) concluded that there is a small but significant effect with 120–240 mg of *Ginkgo biloba* extract on objective measures of cognitive function in Alzheimer's disease. It is likely that there are several mechanisms of action for this herb, which act synergistically, including acting as scavengers for free radicals (DeFeudis 1991). Side-effects associated with *Ginkgo biloba* are rare.

Key point ▶

> Future treatments for Alzheimer's disease may include the use of neural transplantation, vaccination, cholesterol-lowering agents, chelating agents, dietary supplements and herbal remedies.

DEMENTIA OF FRONTAL LOBE TYPE

Dementias of frontal lobe type, where the primary pathology is frontal, present a clinical picture of early personality change, behaviour changes, aphasia and incontinence. There is an absence of Alzheimer's pathology and onset of the dementia is generally earlier than in patients with Alzheimer's disease. **Pick's disease** is characterised by dementia of the frontal lobe type and pathologically by the presence of Pick's bodies, circular cytoplasmic inclusions within neurones. It is much less common than Alzheimer's disease and is more common in females. Pick's disease may be inherited through a single autosomal dominant gene. The disease is progressive and the life expectancy can be anywhere from 2 to 20 years. There is no treatment, although the associated psychiatric symptoms can be treated with psychotropic medicines.

Key point ▶

> Dementias of frontal lobe type, where the primary pathology is frontal, present a clinical picture of early personality change, behaviour changes, aphasia and incontinence.

CORTICAL LEWY BODY DISEASE

Cortical Lewy body disease is responsible for about a fifth of the total cases of dementia in the UK. It is a syndrome characterised by extrapyramidal rigidity and is associated with Lewy body pathology. Lewy bodies are round deposits found in damaged nerve cells but, unlike Alzheimer's pathology, are not associated with plaques and tangles. Lewy bodies are typically found in the substantia nigra in Parkinson's disease but in this type of dementia are scattered throughout the cortex. The presentation of cortical Lewy body disease is often with hallucinations or delusions.

There is no specific treatment for dementia of this type although it has been suggested that people with cortical Lewy body disease may be particularly responsive to the acetylcholinesterase inhibitors **donepezil hydrochloride** and **rivastigmine**.

Cortical Lewy body disease is a syndrome characterised by extrapyramidal rigidity and is associated with Lewy body pathology.

◀ *Key point*

VASCULAR DEMENTIAS

Vascular dementia is a global term for all types of vascular injury that cause cognitive deficits. Formerly known as arteriosclerotic dementia, vascular dementia includes multi-infarct dementia and can be distinguished from dementia in Alzheimer's disease by its history of onset, clinical features and subsequent course. There is usually a history of transient ischaemic attacks (TIAs), resulting in brief impairment of consciousness or temporary paralysis. The dementia may also follow a series of cerebrovascular accidents where memory and thinking can be impaired. Infarction, death of brain tissue as a result of insufficient oxygen and nutrients, causes the dementia and the effect of further infarcts is cumulative. The onset, typically later in life, is usually abrupt and the deterioration stepwise. Many patients have a history of cardiovascular disease, hypertension and diabetes. Smoking increases the risk for vascular dementia. Insight and personality may be well preserved.

Vascular dementia is a global term for all types of vascular injury that cause cognitive deficits. Risk factors include cardiovascular disease, hypertension, diabetes and smoking.

◀ *Key point*

The diagnosis of vascular dementia is made using a detailed clinical history supported by physical assessment, neurological examination and occasionally brain imaging studies. Treatments are not specific to the dementia and largely target underlying medical problems. These include anticoagulants such as aspirin and the control of hypertension and cardiac disease. Despite the widespread use of these treatments – as many as 80% of patients with cognitive impairment are prescribed aspirin – there is little evidence for their effectiveness. A Cochrane Review by Williams *et al.* (2002) concluded that there is no evidence that aspirin is effective in treating patients with a diagnosis of vascular dementia.

DEMENTIA ASSOCIATED WITH ALCOHOL MISUSE

Dementia associated with alcohol misuse can be described as a disorder in which changes of cognition, affect, personality or behaviour are present beyond the period when alcohol might reasonably be having a direct effect (i.e. beyond the period of acute intoxication). It should be distinguished from the effects of alcohol withdrawal. This type of dementia occurs after prolonged, sustained drinking, likely to be in excess of 15 years, and is not exclusively found in the elderly.

Dementia associated with alcohol misuse is caused by a combination of the direct toxic effects of alcohol on the neurones and nutritional deficiencies, such as thiamine (vitamin B_1), related to the alcohol misuse. The clinical presentation is not dissimilar to that of other dementias such as Alzheimer's disease. Treatment should include abstinence from alcohol and adequate nutrition and vitamin supplementation. Secondary health problems, such as cirrhosis, should also be treated.

Key point ▶

> Dementia associated with alcohol misuse is caused by a combination of the direct toxic effects of alcohol on the neurones and nutritional deficiencies, such as thiamine (vitamin B_1), related to the alcohol misuse.

HUNTINGTON'S DISEASE

Huntington's disease is an inherited neurodegenerative disorder that affects around 6000 people in the UK and results in generalised cerebral atrophy. It tends to develop in people in mid-life, though not exclusively, and over a period of some 15–20 years it produces movement disorders, psychiatric disturbance, dementia and eventual death. The core pathology involves a degeneration of the basal ganglia. The loss of neurones leads to the development of a range of symptoms for which there is no cure. Treatments aim to replace depleted neurotransmitters and can help in the early stages of the disease. However, they ultimately fail as the progressive loss of neurones continues. The clinical and pathological aspects of Huntington's disease make it a candidate for curative neural transplant therapies. Barker and Rosser (2001) have reviewed neural transplantation therapies for Huntington's disease and conclude that major practical and ethical problems still confront the field. However, there may still be a future for curative cell therapies as the tools for manipulating and growing cells develop.

Key point ▶

> Huntington's disease is an inherited neurodegenerative disorder that tends to develop in people in midlife. Over a period of some 15-20 years it produces movement disorders, psychiatric disturbance, dementia and eventual death.

A single autosomal dominant gene, mapped to the short arm of chromosome 4, causes Huntington's disease. It is inherited equally by men and women and is present in about 1 in 14 000 people in the UK. Since the faulty gene is dominant it does not skip generations and produces a 50% chance of offspring inheriting the gene when born to an affected parent. The late onset of the disease often means which couples have to make difficult decisions when considering raising a family. Screening for Huntington's disease has been available since 1993 and is offered alongside counselling and psychological support.

The early symptoms of Huntington's disease include slight unsteadiness and clumsiness. The movement disorders, as they become more pronounced, give rise to chorea. This is involuntary movement that develops in response to imbalances of dopamine in the brain. Huntington's disease is also known as Huntington's chorea for this very reason. A subtle change in personality, evident in the early stages, develops into dementia in which cognitive function is severely affected. Psychiatric symptoms such as psychosis and depression are common.

DELIRIUM

Delirium is a reversible confusional state where the symptoms appear rapidly, over hours or days, and fluctuate greatly. Symptoms include altered consciousness, cognitive impairment, psychiatric symptoms and autonomic changes, producing a high mortality and morbidity. The presence of dementia increases the susceptibility to developing delirium.

> Delirium is a reversible confusional state where the symptoms appear rapidly, over hours or days, and fluctuate greatly.

◀ *Key point*

Delirium is probably more common than figures suggest. For instance, the symptoms of delirium are very similar to those of dementia and often the only indication of its existence is a sudden increase in irritability or disturbance of the sleep–wake cycle. It is probable that delirium exists, undetected, in many people with dementia.

It is important to detect and treat any underlying conditions that are contributing to the mental state of a patient. These are generally systemic illnesses although adverse effects of drugs, particularly the direct anticholinergic effect of prescribed medications, are among the most common causes of delirium in older patients. The pharmacological management of the psychiatric symptoms of delirium should take account of this. High-potency antipsychotics, such as haloperidol, have the advantage of producing less orthostatic hypotension, are less sedating and have few anticholinergic side-effects.

SUMMARY

This chapter has introduced the reader to the concept of dementia. The clinical picture of dementia has been explored in relation to the leading theories for the aetiology of the pathological changes associated with a range of dementias. Treatment options, particularly the role of acetyl-cholinesterases in the treatment of Alzheimer's disease, have been reviewed.

REFERENCES AND FURTHER READING

Alzheimer's Disease International (2002) *Alzheimer's Disease International* [online]. ADI, London. http://www.alz.co.uk/

Alzheimer's Society (2000) *Appraisal of the Drugs for Alzheimer's Disease*. Alzheimer's Society, London.

Barker, R.A. and Rosser, A.E. (2001) Neural transplantation therapies for Parkinson's and Huntington's diseases. *Drug Discovery Today*, 6, 575–582.

Benson, D.F. (1994) *The Neurology of Thinking*. Oxford University Press, Oxford.

Birks, J.S., Melzer, D. and Beppu, H. (2002a) Donepezil for mild and moderate Alzheimer's disease (Cochrane Review). In: *The Cochrane Library*, issue 1. Update Software, Oxford.

Birks, J.S., Grimley Evans, J., Iakovidou, V. and Tsolaki, M. (2002b) Rivastigmine for Alzheimer's disease (Cochrane Review). In: *The Cochrane Library*, issue 1. Update Software, Oxford.

Craddock, N. and Lendon, C. (1998) New susceptibility gene for Alzheimer's disease on chromosome 12? *Lancet*, 352, 1720–1721.

DeFeudis, F.V. (1991) *Ginkgo Biloba Extract (Egb 761): Pharmacological Activities and Clinical Applications*. Elsevier, New York.

Dorrell, S. (2001) Alzheimer's disease – a metallic problem. *Drug Discovery Today*, 6, 61–62.

Georgotas, A., McCue, E. and Cooper, T.B. (1989) A placebo-controlled comparison of nortriptyline and phenelzine in maintenance therapy of elderly depressed patients. *Archives of General Psychiatry*, 46, 783–786.

Golde, T.E. and Eckman, C.B. (2001) Cholesterol modulation as an emerging strategy for the treatment of Alzheimer's disease. *Drug Discovery Today*, 6, 1049–1055.

Habeck, M. (2001) Is Alzheimer's disease a form of cancer? *Drug Discovery Today*, 6, 651–652.

Higgins, J.P.T. and Flicker, L. (2002) Lecithin for dementia and cognitive impairment (Cochrane Review) In: *The Cochrane Library*, issue 1. Update Software, Oxford.

Katzman, R. (2000) Epidemiology of Alzheimer's disease. *Neurobiology of Aging*, 21, S1.

Kay, D.W.K., Foster, E.M., McKechnie, A.A. and Roth, M. (1970) Mental illness and hospital use in the elderly: a random sample followed up. *Comprehensive Psychiatry*, 11, 26–35.

Kilpatrick, C., Burns, R. and Blumbergs, P.C. (1983) Identical twins with Alzheimer's disease. *Journal of Neurology, Neurosurgery and Psychiatry*, 46, 421–425.

Kirchner, V., Kelly, C.A. and Harvey, R.J. (2002) Thioridazine for dementia (Cochrane Review). In: *The Cochrane Library*, issue 1. Update Software, Oxford.

Kopelman, M.D. (1985) Rates of forgetting in Alzheimer-type dementia and Korsakoff's syndrome. *Neuropsychologia*, 23, 623–638.

Lishman, A. (1987) *Organic Psychiatry*, 2nd edn. Blackwell, Oxford.

Lonergan, E., Luxenberg, J. and Colford, J. (2002) Haloperidol for agitation in dementia (Cochrane Review). In: *The Cochrane Library*, issue 1. Update Software, Oxford.

Lopez-Arrieta, J.M., Rodriguez, J.L. and Sanz, F. (2002) Efficacy and safety of nicotine on Alzheimer's disease patients (Cochrane Review). In: *The Cochrane Library*, issue 1. Update Software, Oxford.

Department of Health (2001) *National Service Framework for Older People*. The Stationery Office, London.

Oken, B.S., Storzbach, D.M. and Kaye, J.A. (1998) The efficacy of *Ginkgo biloba* on cognitive function in Alzheimer disease. *Archives of Neurology*, 55, 1409–1415.

Olin, J. and Schneider, L. (2002) Galantamine for Alzheimer's disease (Cochrane Review). In: *The Cochrane Library*, issue 1. Update Software, Oxford.

Owens, J. (2001) Milking nature for Alzheimer's treatment. Drug Discovery Today 6, 17, 866–868.

Ray, W. (1992) Psychotropic drugs and injuries among the elderly: a review. *Journal of Clinical Psychopharmacology* 12, 386–396.

Schenk, D. (1999) Immunization with amyloid-beta attenuates Alzheimer-disease-like pathology in the PDAPP mouse. *Nature*, **400**, 173–177.

Tabet, N., Birks, J., Grimley Evans, J. *et al.* (2002) Vitamin E for Alzheimer's disease (Cochrane Review). In: *The Cochrane Library*, issue 1. Update Software, Oxford.

Taylor, D., McConnell, D., McConnell, H. and Kerwin, R. (2001) *The South London and Maudsley NHS Trust 2001 Prescribing Guidelines*, 6th Edition. Martin Dunitz, London.

Williams, P.S., Rands, G., Orrel, M. and Spector, A. (2002) Aspirin for vascular dementia (Cochrane Review). In: *The Cochrane Library*, issue 1. Update Software, Oxford.

SELF-TEST QUESTIONS

1. Impairment in which of the following areas is the most common symptom of dementia?
   a. memory
   b. thinking
   c. orientation
   d. language

2. Which of the following terms used to describe the cognitive deficits experienced by someone with dementia refers to the loss of the ability to perform previously learned motor tasks?
   a. amnesia
   b. aphasia
   c. apraxia
   d. agnosia

3. The defining microscopic features in the brains of people with Alzheimer's disease are:
   a. a reduction in gyri and widening of sulci
   b. the presence of neuritic plaques and neurofibrillary tangles
   c. atrophy in the brain stem
   d. all of the above

4. Neuritic plaques are extracellular lesions with beta-amyloid deposits, formed from the abnormal processes of neurones. True or false?

5. The amyloid cascade hypothesis of Alzheimer's disease theorises that:

a. the disease is caused by the excessive presence of beta-amyloid, leading to the destruction of neurones

b. the production of APP may be compromised by a genetic abnormality that leads to the formation of beta-amyloid deposits and ultimately plaques and tangles

c. Apo-E may be unable to properly bind with and remove beta-amyloid, resulting in its build-up and ultimate destruction of neurones

d. all of the above

6. Which neurotransmitter is believed to play a role in many of the behaviours associated with Alzheimer's disease, particularly those of attention and memory?

a. dopamine

b. acetylcholine

c. serotonin

d. noradrenaline (epinephrine)

7. The neurodegeneration seen in Alzheimer's disease may be caused through excitotoxicity produced at the NMDA glutamate receptor. True or false?

8. Donepezil hydrochloride, a drug used in the treatment of Alzheimer's disease, works by:

a. blocking dopamine receptors in the mesolimbic dopamine pathway

b. enhancing the effect of GABA at its receptor complex

c. blocking acetylcholinesterase in cholinergic pathways

d. increasing neurotransmission in the serotonergic pathways

9. Rivastigmine is less beneficial for people with mild to moderate Alzheimer's disease than those with more progressed symptoms. True or false?

10. Dementias of frontal lobe type are characterised by:

a. disordered movement

b. behavioural and personality disturbance

c. late onset

d. none of the above

11. Delirium can be distinguished from dementia in that delirium is associated with:

a. slow insidious onset

b. erratic, fluctuating behaviour

c. memory loss

d. poor social judgement

12. The treatment of delirium consists mainly of:

a. identifying and treating the underlying cause

b. prescribing acetylcholinesterase inhibitors

c. reality orientation

d. all of the above

SUBSTANCE MISUSE

INTRODUCTION

Previous chapters have addressed the use of psychotropic drugs for therapeutic purposes. The aim here is to explore the nature of substance misuse. The term 'substance' is preferred to 'drug' as many substances of misuse are naturally occurring, or were not intended for use by humans. The misuse of substances creates a major health problem throughout the world and provides a heavy medical, psychiatric and social burden to society. This chapter will begin by giving some explanation of the terms used in relation to substance misuse. The psychopharmacology of reward will provide the basis for discussing a range of commonly misused substances and their effects on the brain when used in the short and long term.

Substance misuse

The acceptable use of substances is generally defined by cultures and therefore differs from one culture to another and within one culture over time. When the use of a substance falls outside culturally approved boundaries and leads to adverse consequences it is deemed misuse. This chapter will examine the effect of repeated self-administration of substances on the brain. Substances of misuse have, by their very nature, reinforcing properties; in other words, they produce pleasure that leads to repeated use. The reinforcing properties of substances of misuse cause neurochemical changes in the brain during intoxication, affecting behaviour and producing psychological distress.

> The acceptable use of substances is generally defined by cultures and therefore differs from one culture to another and within one culture over time.

◀ **Key point**

Dependence and withdrawal

Dependence is produced when the repeated administration of a substance with reinforcing properties causes a physiological state of neuroadaptation and the cessation of its administration leads to a withdrawal syndrome.

Dependence, according to the World Health Organization's International Classification of Diseases (ICD-10), is a syndrome manifested by three or more of the following, experienced at some time during the same 12-month period:

- A strong desire to use the substance
- Problems controlling the use of the substance
- The presence of a withdrawal syndrome on cessation of the use of the substance
- The development of tolerance to the substance, producing a need for increased amounts of the substance to achieve the desired effect or a reduced effect with continued use of the same amount of the substance
- Loss of interest in activities other than those necessary to obtain the substance or recover from its effects
- Continued use of the substance despite an awareness of the harm this may cause.

It is important to make a distinction between the terms 'dependence' and 'addiction'. Addiction is not defined in psychopharmacology and its use should be confined to the behavioural aspects of substance misuse rather than the physiological state of neuroadaptation. Many commonly used medications produce dependence. The abrupt cessation of these medications may lead to a relapse of the disorder or produce symptoms worse than the original condition, a phenomenon known as **rebound**. We would not consider, however, that the person is addicted to their medication, although they are physiologically dependent on it. Rebound is distinct from withdrawal and involves psychological and physiological reactions to abrupt discontinuation of a tolerance-producing drug. **Withdrawal** is characterised by symptoms such as craving and sympathetic nervous system overactivity.

The discontinuation of a dependence-producing substance without the production of a withdrawal syndrome requires **detoxification**. This is achieved either by slowly withdrawing the dependence-producing substance itself or a substituted cross-dependent substance with a similar pharmacological mechanism of action. The neurones of the brain can then readapt without producing the symptoms of withdrawal. It may also be necessary to slowly withdraw medications that are likely to produce rebound. This is known as **tapered discontinuation**.

Addiction can be described as a syndrome characterised by compulsive substance-seeking behaviour that results in impairment in social and psychological functions or damage to health. Tolerance and physical dependence are not the core of addiction. If they were, treatment for addiction would simply consist of detoxification. The urge to continue or resume substance-taking behaviour continues after detoxification and long periods of abstinence, leading to high rates of relapse. High relapse rates are based on changes in brain function that continue for months or years after the last use of a substance, and their interaction with environmental factors such as stress and situational triggers.

Key point ▶

> Addiction can be described as a syndrome characterised by compulsive substance-seeking behaviour that results in impairment in social and psychological functions or damage to health.

Addictive disorders commonly exist alongside psychiatric disorders, including anxiety disorders, affective disorders and psychotic disorders. The prevalence of 'dual diagnosis' is higher than can be accounted for by chance overlap (Kessler *et al.*, 1996). One explanation for the presence of dual diagnosis is that a pre-existing psychiatric disorder could lead to an increased likelihood of substance misuse as an attempt to self-medicate psychiatric symptoms (Khantzian, 1985). Alternatively, substance misuse could produce changes in the brain and in social interactions that trigger the development of psychiatric disorders. Schuckit *et al.* (1997) found that many of the psychiatric symptoms associated with addictive disorders begin after the misuse of substances and are resolved simply by abstinence.

Addictive disorders commonly exist alongside psychiatric disorders.

◀ **Key point**

THE PSYCHOPHARMACOLOGY OF REWARD

We have all experienced the feeling of reward that comes with competing in sports, academic achievement or sexual gratification. These are the natural 'highs' that make these experiences pleasurable. It is hypothesised that our reward comes from the stimulation of the mesolimbic dopamine pathway that projects from the midbrain to the limbic system (Figure 7.1). A range of naturally occurring substances including the endorphins, anandamide, acetylcholine and dopamine mediate these highs.

This pathway, however, is thought to be involved not only in the sensation of pleasure but also the euphoria associated with substance misuse, and the delusions and hallucinations of psychosis. Substances of misuse stimulate the pathway in much the same way as their naturally occurring counterparts, only more powerfully. Opioids act as endor-

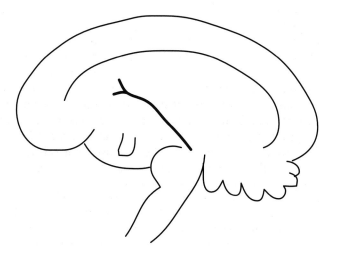

Figure 7.1

Mesolimbic dopamine pathway

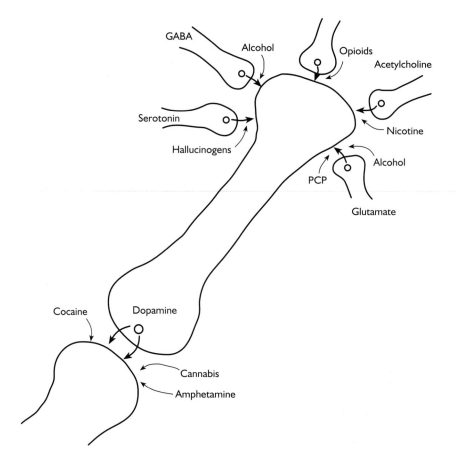

Figure 7.2

Drug interactions with the mesolimbic dopamine pathway

phins, marijuana as anandamide, nicotine as acetylcholine, and cocaine and amphetamine (amfetamine) as dopamine (Figure 7.2). Hence, intense 'highs' can be achieved quickly and effortlessly through the use of such substances. The excessive stimulation of the mesolimbic dopamine pathway comes at a price, however. When the effects subside, postsynaptic receptors crave more of these substances to boost dopamine levels, creating a strong and sometimes overpowering desire for the individual to seek more.

Key point ▶

> The mesolimbic dopamine pathway is thought to be involved not only in the sensation of pleasure but also the euphoria associated with substance misuse and the delusions and hallucinations of psychosis.

It is postulated that there is an optimal range of dopamine receptor stimulation required in the mesolimbic pathway to produce reinforcement. This idea has been used to explain the varied response individuals have to substances of misuse. Those who have few receptors for a particular substance have only a limited initial 'high' but gain greater reward as the dose increases. This could be interpreted as a dysfunctional reward system predisposing these individuals to seek ways of overcoming the problem, namely substance misuse. For individuals with many receptors the initial overwhelming response is likely to lead to an avoidance of the substance in the future. This is given credence by several studies that show which a low initial response to a substance produces a greater risk of later misuse, and *vice versa*.

A low initial response to a substance produces a greater risk of later misuse.

◀ **Key point**

ALCOHOL

Alcohol is the most widely used substance in the UK. Most people drink alcohol, the majority without problems. However, misuse of alcohol is associated with a diverse range of health, social and legal problems. Binge drinkers are at greater risk when operating machinery, including driving cars, and form a significant proportion of those involved in accidents. They are also more likely to exhibit violent behaviour. Longer-term use is likely to lead to increasing health, social and legal problems. The cost to society, including the impact this has on the National Health Service, has been estimated in a number of studies (Maynard and Godfrey, 1994).

Alcohol misuse is common, although the number of people with unrecognised problems makes it very difficult to estimate how many are involved. There is a positive correlation between risk and the amount of alcohol consumed. Alcohol consumption is measured in units of alcohol. One unit contains about 10 g of alcohol and is defined as half a pint of beer, a glass of wine or a standard pub measure of spirits. Most people drinking in their own homes pour more than standard measures, beers are becoming stronger and the introduction to the market of alcopops makes it very difficult to work out how much alcohol is being consumed.

The introduction of a sliding scale of weekly units of alcohol defined risk as increasing above 14 units for women and 21 units for men (Royal College of Psychiatrists, 1986). Levels above 36 units a week for women and 51 units a week for men are likely to cause problems. This system does not take account of binge drinking within the week. Daily levels would be a more useful guide.

A study by Bennett *et al.* (1996) looked at the proportion of the population drinking at different levels. They found which a significant number of people drink at very high levels. Young males below the age of 30 years are the most highly represented group at higher levels. Single and separated men and women are at greater risk of problem drinking than those in other groups (Meltzer *et al.*, 1995).

Key point ▶

There is a positive correlation between risk and the amount of alcohol consumed.

The pharmacological and toxic effects of alcohol lead to a wide range of physical and psychological problems, not just for people who are alcohol-dependent but also for people who binge-drink. A study by Chick (1994) revealed that 15–30% of male and 8–15% of female admissions to general hospitals in the UK had alcohol-related problems. The most commonly encountered problems are gastrointestinal, cardiovascular, neurological and neuropsychiatric. Alcohol is the biggest cause of liver damage in the UK. Excessive alcohol consumption is also a significant risk factor for cardiovascular disease, including alcohol-related hypertension. There is, however, a slightly higher risk of coronary heart disease in non-drinkers compared with light or moderate drinkers, suggesting that alcohol in moderate amounts has a protective effect.

Heavy alcohol consumption can lead to dietary neglect (deficiencies in thiamine) and toxicity produced by the alcohol and its metabolite acetaldehyde. Neuropsychiatric disorders such as Wernicke's encephalopathy may ensue. Wernicke's encephalopathy responds to parenteral **thiamine** but, if untreated, it progresses to Korsakoff's syndrome, in which short-term memory and orientation are affected. Korsakoff's syndrome does not generally respond to thiamine.

The incidence of alcohol problems and that of psychiatric disorders are both high. It is not surprising, therefore, that the likelihood of a patient with an alcohol problem having a comorbid psychiatric disorder is also high. There are many psychiatric complications of heavy drinking and many psychiatric disorders associated with heavy drinking. Alcohol-related hallucinatory states include transient hallucinations, delirium tremens (DTs) and alcoholic hallucinosis. Transient hallucinations may be a precursor to the onset of DTs and alcoholic hallucinosis.

Delirium tremens is a toxic confusional state resulting from alcohol withdrawal in a patient who tends to have a long history of alcohol dependence. It is short-lived, commonly lasting for 3–5 days. The symptoms, including clouding of consciousness and confusion, hallucinations, delusions, agitation and tremor, tend to peak between 72 and 96 hours from the time of the last drink (Naranjo and Sellers 1986). The condition normally shows gradual improvement but is fatal in about 5% of cases (Chick 1989). Skullcap (*Scutellaria laterifolia*), a member of the mint family, Labatiae, is a herbal treatment shown to have efficacy for delirium tremens (Newall *et al.*, 1996).

Key point ▶

Delirium tremens is a toxic confusional state resulting from alcohol withdrawal in a patient who tends to have a long history of alcohol dependence.

Alcoholic hallucinosis occurs during or after a period of heavy alcohol consumption. It differs from DTs in that consciousness remains clear. Marked hallucinations are common and are often accompanied by delusions, which attempt to explain the hallucinations. Recovery is slow, usually taking several weeks.

The pharmacological action of alcohol is poorly understood. It has an effect on a wide variety of neurotransmitter systems, leading to confusion as to its mechanism for producing acute intoxication and chronic dependence, tolerance and withdrawal. It is believed to act as an allosteric modulator at gamma-aminobutyric acid (GABA) receptors, enhancing the inhibition produced there, and reduce excitation at the N-methyl-D-aspartate (NMDA) glutamate receptor. Alcohol thus acts as a depressant of neuronal functioning, which may explain to some extent its intoxicating effects.

Alcohol acts as a depressant of neuronal functioning.

◀ *Key point*

The rewarding effect of alcohol may be mediated in part by its effect on GABA and glutamate, which influence dopamine release in the mesolimbic dopamine pathway. There may also be an associated release of opiates and cannabinoids in this system in response to alcohol. **Naltrexone**, an opiate receptor antagonist, blocks opiate receptors, thus removing the opiate-induced pleasure associated with alcohol. It is sometimes used to reduce craving in alcohol-dependent patients and increase abstinence, particularly in the early stages of abstinence when the risk of relapse is highest. A Cochrane Review (Srisurapanont and Jarusuraisin, 2002) concluded that naltrexone has some benefits for patients with alcohol dependence, particularly when administered concurrently with psychosocial treatments.

Naltrexone, an opiate receptor antagonist, is sometimes used to reduce craving in alcohol-dependent patients and support abstinence.

◀ *Key point*

Alcohol withdrawal is associated with significant morbidity and mortality when poorly managed. There is evidence that sensitisation occurs, rendering repeated withdrawals progressively more severe. The treatment of withdrawal symptoms may reduce the sensitisation process (Brown *et al.*, 1988).

The pharmacotherapy for alcohol withdrawal generally involves the use of benzodiazepines. They have become the treatment of choice because they are non-tolerant with alcohol and have anticonvulsant properties. The majority of alcohol-dependent patients undergo detoxification in the community. Depending on the severity of the dependence a typical detoxification regime might be 10–20 mg of **chlordiazepoxide** four times a day, reducing gradually over 5–7 days.

If the dependence is severe, an inpatient protocol may be necessary. This involves a more flexible approach during the first 24 hours whereby the dose of chlordiazepoxide is titrated against the severity of the withdrawal symptoms. The closer monitoring possible in an inpatient setting allows for greater responsiveness and avoidance of both under- and overtreatment, each with associated complications. Nursing observations should include monitoring of blood pressure and pulse and the use of an alcohol withdrawal scale, such as the Addiction Research Foundation Clinical Institute Withdrawal Assessment – Alcohol (CIWA-Ar). This is a valid and reliable 10-item rating scale that is a useful guide for clinical interventions. Mayo-Smith (1997) gives guidance for the pharmacological management of alcohol withdrawal.

Key point ▶

> Alcohol withdrawal is associated with significant morbidity and mortality when poorly managed.

A potentially fatal consequence of alcohol withdrawal is the alcohol withdrawal syndrome. This can develop within hours of their last drink in patients who are dependent on alcohol. When the alcohol level in the blood suddenly drops the brain, which is used to the constant presence of alcohol, remains hyperexcited, causing the withdrawal syndrome. The signs and symptoms associated with this syndrome can be grouped under the following headings:

- Autonomic nervous system hyperactivity (such as tachycardia, sweating, tremors and general restlessness);
- Neuronal excitation (seizures);
- Delirium tremens (confusion, disorientation, fever and thought and perceptual disturbance).

Claassen and Adinoff (1999) have published guidelines for the management of the alcohol withdrawal syndrome.

Disulfiram is a drug used in the UK in the treatment of chronic alcohol dependence. It is generally offered to patients who aim to abstain from alcohol and have previously failed to do so. It works by blocking the metabolism of alcohol, causing the accumulation of the noxious by-product acetaldehyde. This is so unpleasant that it acts as a deterrent to consuming alcohol while taking disulfiram. The effect is dose-dependent and requires the patient to take the drug regularly. Disulfiram works best when its administration is supervised (Hughes and Cook, 1997). The majority of patients do not like taking this drug and simply do not adhere to the prescription (Fuller *et al.*, 1986). It is only used as an oral preparation in the UK as its release from depot preparations has been found to be unreliable.

Anticraving medications have been introduced to help patients avoid relapsing into alcohol misuse. Naltrexone, an opiate receptor antagonist, has been shown to reduce craving for alcohol and improve relapse rates. Alcohol is less rewarding when opiate receptors are blocked.

Acamprosate, a relatively new medication, appears to reduce the long-lasting neuronal hyperexcitability that follows chronic alcohol use (Putzke *et al.*, 1996). Acamprosate interacts with the NMDA receptor, forming a substitute for the glutamate effect of alcohol during abstinence. It is believed to modify drinking behaviour by reducing the intensity of and response to cues and triggers to drinking and thereby to increase abstinence (Sass *et al.*, 1996; Whitworth *et al.*, 1996). It is recommended that acamprosate is initiated as soon as possible after the withdrawal period and continued for 1 year (Hall and Zador, 1997). It can be continued in the event of a relapse, as it does not interact with alcohol or benzodiazepines.

Alcoholics who start drinking at a very early age are probably the most difficult to treat. They tend to have the most intractable problems, including a high degree of antisocial behaviour, and have a high rate of drop out of treatment. Johnson (2000) has investigated **ondansetron,** which blocks the 5HT3A receptor, for its use in this population. It was found to increase the number of days abstinent by 20% and was even more effective when combined with naltrexone.

CASE STUDY 7.1	FRED, AN ALCOHOLIC

Read this case study and then attempt to answer the questions that follow.

Fred began drinking lager at an early age and, while to begin with he became drunk very quickly, he was soon able to drink much more than his friends. In his desire to become drunk quickly again he turned to strong ciders and spirits. Fred gained the effect he was looking for but, after maintaining this for some time, he began to experience tremors the next morning. He overcame these by having more to drink, until eventually he was drinking pretty much the whole day.

Following a succession of injuries and failed relationships, Fred suddenly decided to stop drinking. The problems he experienced resulted in him returning to alcohol the very same day. He later sought help from an alcohol service and was prescribed a reducing regime of chlordiazepoxide. Fred remained abstinent from alcohol for only a short time until his craving resulted in him drinking once again.

1. Apply the terms intoxication, tolerance, dependence and withdrawal to Fred's case.
2. What part did chlordiazepoxide play in his initial treatment?
3. What alternatives are there for his future treatment?

STIMULANTS

Cocaine is a stimulant that works by blocking monoamine transporters. It may also promote the release of monoamines from the presynaptic neurone. Inhibition of the dopamine transporter in particular produces euphoria, reduces fatigue and increases mental acuity, the property of cocaine that leads to its misuse. However, higher doses of the drug can lead to unwanted effects such as tremor, restlessness, paranoia, panic and stereotyped behaviours. In overdose, heart failure, seizures and stroke can occur.

Key point ▶

> Cocaine is a stimulant that works by blocking monoamine transporters.

Long-term misuse of cocaine tends to produce a downregulation of dopamine receptors as they adapt to the constant presence of the drug. Acute intoxication produces euphoria, which is followed by the 'crash', a period of increasing agitation and anxiety and a craving for more of the drug. If, after several days, no further cocaine is taken, a withdrawal syndrome is likely. This is characterised by a lack of energy and interest and increased craving. This state closely resembles major depression and is in stark contrast to the fantastic highs experienced during acute intoxication. Time alone will allow the dopamine system to return to its previous state, providing the patient is able and willing to remain abstinent.

As well as producing tolerance, cocaine can also produce reverse tolerance, in which the dopamine receptors become sensitised, producing overactivity in the dopamine pathways. This occurs with chronic misuse of cocaine and can produce an acute paranoid psychosis. This is not surprising, given the dopamine hypothesis. The overactivity in the mesolimbic dopamine pathway is not dissimilar to the pathophysiology underlying the positive symptoms of schizophrenia. This psychosis responds to antipsychotic medication.

Key point ▶

> Chronic misuse of cocaine can produce an acute paranoid psychosis.

There are several treatments undergoing investigation for use in people with a cocaine addiction. **Vigabatrin**, an anticonvulsant, has been shown to reduce cocaine-seeking in animals. It works by increasing the levels of GABA, which subsequently reduces levels of dopamine and thus reduces craving for cocaine. **Baclofen** also works on the GABA system by a different mechanism and is being studied for possible use. Vaccines are also under investigation in animals. Immunisation with a cocaine conjugate reduced cocaine-induced stereotyped behaviour in rats (Carrera *et al.*, 1995). The antibodies also reduced the concentration of cocaine in the brains of the rats. A likely problem with the use of such a vaccine is that the antibodies could be overwhelmed by a high dose of cocaine or the cocaine could be replaced by another stimulant.

Amphetamines, particularly D-amfetamine and methamfetamine, are also stimulants of the dopamine pathways. They work by promoting the release of dopamine at the synapse, producing effects similar to those seen with cocaine misuse. The 'high' produced with amphetamines is longer-lasting but less intense than that experienced with cocaine but other than that the effects are similar. Amfetamine is a drug with strong reinforcing properties, producing a high potential for relapse (Schuckit, 1994). Detoxification and rehabilitation programmes work in only 20–40% of cases, as measured by continued abstinence and fewer life problems in the subsequent year (Meyer, 1992).

> Amphetamines work by promoting the release of dopamine at the synapse, thus producing effects similar to those seen with cocaine misuse.

HALLUCINOGENS

The hallucinogens include drugs such as D-lysergic acid diethylamide (LSD), mescaline and the synthetically produced 3,4-methylenedioxymethamfetamine (MDMA), also known as 'Ecstasy' because of the subjective state produced by its use. The 'trip' they produce during intoxication can include visual illusions and hallucinations, experienced in clear consciousness, and enhanced awareness of both external and internal stimuli. The subjective, psychedelic experience is often described as an expansion of the mind and can be interpreted as a religious experience. Sometimes the user will experience 'a bad trip', which has all the symptoms of a panic attack. Another problem associated with the hallucinogens is the possibility of the user experiencing 'flashbacks'. This is a poorly understood phenomenon where the user experiences a spontaneous reoccurrence of some symptoms that occurred during intoxication. The flashbacks, lasting from a few seconds to several hours, occur in the absence of the drug, possibly even months after the drug was last used, and may be triggered by a range of environmental stimuli.

> Some users of hallucinogens experience a phenomenon known as 'flashbacks'.

CANNABIS

Cannabis can have both stimulant and sedative effects. Intoxication is associated with a feeling of relaxation and there may be a slowing of thought processes and short-term memory disturbance. At relatively low doses visual and auditory distortions can occur. Cardiovascular effects include increased heart rate and lowered blood pressure. There is also evidence for an acute toxic psychosis produced by cannabis. Higher doses can induce panic and confusion and mood changes may progress to feelings of depersonalisation and loss of insight. Visual and auditory hallucinations may be present. While some have argued for the existence of a chronic psychosis (Chopra and Smith, 1974), others believe this to be chronic intoxication (cannabis has a long half-life).

Cannabis preparations have, as their psychoactive substances, cannabinoids, the main one being delta-9-tetrahydrocannabinoid (THC). Isbell *et al.* (1967) demonstrated that the psychomimetic effects (mimicking a state of psychosis) of cannabis were dose dependent. It is important to note, therefore, the relative amount of THC in different preparations. Infusions may contain 1–10% THC, as may the marijuana 'reefer', while hashish is likely to have 8–15% THC. A level as high as 60% THC can be found in hashish oil extracted from the resin. It is also worth noting that acute use of cannabis can be detected in urine for at least a week following its administration, while chronic use is likely to produce a positive result for 4 weeks or more (Garrett, 1979).

Key point ▶

> Cannabinoids are the psychoactive substances found in cannabis preparations.

NICOTINE

Cigarette smoking delivers carcinogens and other toxins to the body, which damage the heart and lungs and other tissues. However, in terms of psychopharmacology, the main substance of interest is nicotine. Nicotine binds with nicotinic cholinergic receptors, producing reinforcement as a result of stimulation of the mesolimbic dopamine pathway. Hence, smokers have a sense of reward, including enhanced cognition and elevation of mood. The mechanism of action is similar to that seen with cocaine and amphetamines except that the 'rush' is much less intense and declines only slowly. The effects on behaviour are thus much more subtle.

Key point ▶

> Nicotine in cigarette smoke binds with nicotinic cholinergic receptors, producing reinforcement as a result of stimulation of the mesolimbic dopamine pathway.

Nicotine is able to produce dependence and withdrawal. The nicotine withdrawal syndrome is characterised by agitation and craving and is particularly troublesome for people wanting to detoxify. A range of nicotine replacement therapies for smoking cessation have been introduced, including nicotine gum, nicotine transdermal patch, nicotine nasal spray, nicotine inhaler and nicotine sublingual tablets. A Cochrane Review (Silagy *et al.*, 2002) concluded that they are all effective as part of a strategy to promote smoking cessation, increasing quit rates by a factor of approximately 1.5–2.

The nicotine replacement therapies are able to deliver a supply of nicotine, allowing the dopamine receptors to gradually readapt, thus avoiding the withdrawal syndrome. The dose of nicotine supplied through the various therapies can be reduced slowly on a time course tolerable to the individual. The effectiveness of the nicotine replacement therapies is largely independent of the intensity of additional support provided to the smoker (Silagy *et al.*, 2002) although they are dependent on the motivation of the smoker to quit. Nicotine replacement therapy can also be used for several months following detoxification as a maintenance treatment to block craving and improve the likelihood of continued abstinence (Fiore *et al.*, 1994).

Nicotine replacement therapies are able to deliver a supply of nicotine, allowing the dopamine receptors to gradually readapt, thus avoiding the withdrawal syndrome.

◄ **Key point**

There is promising evidence that the dopamine and noradrenaline (norepinephrine) reuptake inhibitor **bupropion** may be more effective than nicotine replacement therapy in reducing the craving that occurs during abstinence (Silagy *et al.*, 2002). Bupropion is an antidepressant that reduces craving for nicotine and may help in preventing relapse even in the absence of depressive symptoms. Further study is required before bupropion becomes accepted for use in this way. **Clonidine** has also been used to reduce the withdrawal symptoms associated with nicotine use. A Cochrane Review conducted by Gourlay *et al.* (2002) concluded that clonidine is effective in promoting smoking cessation, although its prominent side-effects limit its usefulness.

An alternative approach to smoking cessation is the use of nicotine antagonists. **Mecamylamine** is a nicotine antagonist that may reduce the rewarding effect of nicotine and thus reduce the urge to smoke. A Cochrane Review by Lancaster and Stead (2002) tentatively concluded that nicotine and mecamylamine might be superior to nicotine alone in promoting smoking cessation. Rose *et al.* (1994) hypothesised that binding with both an agonist and an antagonist would be more effective and produce less side-effects.

OPIOIDS

Opium has been used for thousands of years as an analgesic and to induce sleep and reports of it being used for its euphoric effects are not uncommon. Opium is derived from the poppy. Any drug derived from this plant, including morphine and codeine, are termed opiates. The term opioid encompasses drugs that have morphine-like activity; they may be natural or synthetic. The synthetically produced **methadone**, like **morphine**, is an opioid. The brain seemingly makes its own endogenous opioids although their number and function are largely unknown. What is clear is that these endogenous opioids are agonists at a variety of receptors, the three most important subtypes being the mu, delta and kappa opioid receptors. The exogenous opioids, including morphine, **codeine** and **heroin**, are also agonists at these same receptors, particularly the mu receptors. At high doses they induce a 'rush' of euphoria, their main reinforcing property, which is followed by a longer period of tranquillity and eventually drowsiness, mental clouding and apathy. Respiratory depression and coma can result from an overdose of an opioid.

Key point ▶

> Opioids are drugs that have morphine-like activity.

Chronic administration of an opioid produces both tolerance and dependence. Adaptation of the opioid receptors produces a physiological need to take increasingly larger doses to achieve the same rush as previously experienced. The escalating dose required to produce euphoria also becomes ever closer to that of an overdose. A further sign of dependence is the production of a withdrawal syndrome when the effects of the opioid begin to wear off. This is characterised by craving for more opioid, dysphoria and autonomic symptoms such as tachycardia, tremor and sweating. The withdrawal syndrome associated with sudden cessation of opioids is known as 'cold turkey' and is subjectively awful. Hence, the user is driven towards finding the next dose of opioid to avoid the consequences of withdrawal. The adaptation that has occurred at the opioid receptors means the chances of experiencing euphoria are significantly reduced. Hence, the user enters a cycle of alternating periods of withdrawal and periods free from withdrawal without euphoria.

Key point ▶

> Opioid withdrawal, known as 'cold turkey', is characterised by craving for more opioid, dysphoria and autonomic symptoms such as tachycardia, tremor and sweating.

Opioid receptors can readapt in the absence of further opioid use. While the opioid withdrawal syndrome is not life-threatening, it is so unpleasant that detoxification generally requires some form of intervention. One way of managing the withdrawal syndrome is to substitute the opioid being misused with a gradually decreasing dose of a long-acting opioid such as methadone (Mattick and Hall, 1996). Methadone itself has a high dependency potential, and as such, should only be prescribed if opioids are being taken regularly and there is good evidence of opioid dependence. Supervision of methadone taking is preferable, particularly in the early stages of treatment. A Cochrane Review conducted by Amato *et al.* (2002) concluded that methadone does have a role to play in reducing withdrawal severity.

Other options for the management of the acute phase of opioid withdrawal include the use of the alpha-2-adrenergic agonists **clonidine** and **lofexidine**. They are particularly effective in reducing the large adrenergic component of opioid withdrawal and have been used in conjunction with opioid antagonists such as naltrexone. Further study is required to assess the effectiveness of a **naltrexone–clonidine combination** for the management of opioid withdrawal (Gowing *et al.*,

2002a). **Buprenorphine** is an opioid that has mixed effects on opioid receptors. At lower doses it acts as an agonist in a similar way to methadone, while at higher doses it becomes an antagonist like naltrexone. A Cochrane Review by Gowing *et al.* (2002b) concluded that buprenorphine has the potential as a medication to ameliorate the signs and symptoms of withdrawal from opioids.

Methadone should only be prescribed if opioids are being taken regularly and there is good evidence of opioid dependence.

◀ **Key point**

The long-term treatment of opioid dependence makes use of both agonist and antagonist medications. **Methadone** is a cross-tolerant slow-onset, long-acting mu opioid receptor agonist that reduces the craving for opioids and largely eliminates the euphoria associated with using a short-acting opioid such as heroin. Patients can be maintained on methadone for many years. Alternatively, patients can be maintained on buprenorphine. As a partial agonist it has limited opioid effects but reduces the effects of other opioids taken concurrently, thereby reducing the likelihood of their use.

Methadone is a cross-tolerant, slow-onset, long-acting mu opioid receptor agonist that reduces the craving for opioids and largely eliminates the euphoria associated with using a short-acting opioid such as heroin.

◀ **Key point**

The antagonists have a high affinity for opioid receptors without producing the effects associated with the opioids. Naltrexone has a particularly high affinity for the mu opioid receptors and no agonist activity (Raynor *et al.*, 1994). It was first introduced in the belief that it would provide an effective treatment for opioid dependence by blocking the effects of opioids taken at the same time. This optimism was short-lived, users preferring the mild opioid-reinforcing effects associated with methadone. Compliance with taking an antagonist such as naltrexone can also be a problem.

BENZODIAZEPINES

Benzodiazepines are drugs that are used predominantly in the treatment of anxiety. Their anxiolytic effects are mediated at the $GABA_A$ receptor complex, where they act as allosteric modulators, enhancing the influx of chloride into the cell and inhibiting its neurotransmission. The interaction of benzodiazepines with their receptors also produces the reinforcing properties of euphoria, tranquillity and sedation that may lead to the misuse of these drugs.

Key point ▶

> Both the anxiolytic effects and reinforcing properties of benzodiaze-pines are mediated at the $GABA_A$ receptor complex, where they act as allosteric modulators, enhancing the influx of chloride into the cell and inhibiting its neurotransmission.

The chronic use of benzodiazepines desensitises their receptors and reduces the ability of the drug to modulate the ion channel. This dependence is likely even following only therapeutic dosages (Greenblatt *et al.*, 1990). Tolerance of benzodiazepines necessitates an increase in dose to induce euphoria and tranquillity and a sudden cessation produces a withdrawal syndrome characterised by severe irritability and anxiety, muscle tension, insomnia and occasional seizures (Davidson 1997). These symptoms are in stark contrast to the acute effects of the drugs and can be relieved by reintroducing a benzodiazepine or allowing the receptors to readapt. A typical detoxification regime would involve a tapered withdrawal of the drug.

Summary

This chapter has introduced substance misuse by giving some explanation of dependence and withdrawal and how they manifest in an individual. The mesolimbic dopamine system has been cited as a possible pathway for the generation of reward and related to the mechanism of action of a range of substances that are commonly misused, including alcohol, stimulants, hallucinogens, cannabis, nicotine, opioids and benzodiazepines. A range of treatments for the management of dependence and withdrawal has been discussed.

References and further reading

Amato, L., Davoli, M., Ferri, M. and Ali, R. (2002) Methadone at tapered doses for the management of opioid withdrawal (Cochrane Review). In: *The Cochrane Library*, issue 1. Update Software, Oxford.

Bennett, N., Jarvis, L., Rowlands, O. *et al.* (1996) *Living in Britain: Results from the 1994 General Household Survey*. HMSO, London.

Brown, M.E., Anton, R.F., Malcolm. R. and Ballenger, J.C. (1988) Alcohol detoxification and withdrawal seizures: clinical support for a kindling hypothesis. *Biological Psychiatry*, **23**, 507–514.

Carrera, M.R., Ashley, J.A., Parsons, L.H. *et al.* (1995) Suppression of psychoactive effects of cocaine by active immunization. *Nature*, **378**, 727–730.

Chick, J. (1989) Delirium tremens. *British Medical Journal*, **298**, 3–4.

Chick, J. (1994) Alcohol problems in the general hospital. *British Medical Bulletin*, **50**, 200–210.

Chopra, G.S. and Smith, J.W. (1974) Psychotic reactions following cannabis use in East Indians. *Archives of General Psychiatry*, **30**, 24–27.

Claassen, C.A. and Adinoff, B. (1999) Alcohol withdrawal syndrome: guidelines for management. *CNS Drugs*, **12**, 279–291.

Davidson, J.R.T. (1997) Use of benzodiazepines in panic disorder. *Journal of Clinical Psychiatry*, **58**(Suppl. 2), 26–28.

Fiore, M.C., Smith, S.S., Jorenby, D.E. and Baker, T.B. (1994) The effectiveness of the nicotine patch for smoking cessation. A meta-analysis. *Journal of the American Medical Association*, **271**, 1940-1947.

Fuller, R.K., Branchey, L., Brightwell, D.R. *et al.* (1986) Disulfiram treatment of alcoholism. A Veterans Administration cooperative study. *Journal of the American Medical Association*, **256**, 1449–1455.

Garrett, E.R. (1979) Pharmacokinetics and disposition of delta (9) tetrahydrocannabinol and its metabolites. In: *Marijuana: Biological Effects* (ed. C.G. Nahas and W.M. Pahon). Pergamon Press, Elmford, NY, pp. 105–121.

Gourlay, S.G., Stead, L.F. and Benowitz, N.L. (2002) Clonidine for smoking cessation (Cochrane Review). In: *The Cochrane Library*, issue 1. Update Software, Oxford.

Gowing, L., Ali, R. and White, J. (2002a) Opioid antagonists and adrenergic agonists for the management of opioid withdrawal (Cochrane Review). In: *The Cochrane Library*, issue 1. Update Software, Oxford.

Gowing, L., Ali, R. and White, J. (2002b) Buprenorphine for the management of opioid withdrawal (Cochrane Review). In: *The Cochrane Library*, issue 1. Update Software, Oxford.

Greenblatt, D.J., Miller, L.G. and Shader, R.L. (1990) Benzodiazepine discontinuation syndromes. *Journal of Psychiatric Research*, **24**(Suppl. 2), 73–80.

Hall, W. and Zador, D. (1997) The alcohol withdrawal syndrome. *The Lancet*, **349**, 1897–1900.

Hughes, J.C. and Cook, C.H. (1997) The efficacy of disulfiram: a review of outcome studies. *Addiction*, **92**, 381–395.

Isbell, H., Gerodetzsky, C.W. and Janiski, D. (1967) Effects of delta-9-trans tetrahydrocannabinoid in man. *Psychopharmacologia*, **11**, 184–188.

Johnson, B.A., Roache, J.D., Javors, M.A. *et al.* (2000) Ondansetron for reduction of drinking among predisposed alcoholic patients. *Journal of the American Medical Association*, **284**, 963–971.

Kessler, R.C., Nelson, C.B., McGonagle, K.A. *et al.* (1996) The epidemiology of co-occurring addictive and mental disorders: implications for prevention and service utilization. *American Journal of Orthopsychiatry*, **66**,17–31.

Khantzian, E.J. (1985) The self-medication hypothesis of addictive disorders: focus on heroin and cocaine dependence. *American Journal of Psychiatry*, **142**, 1259–1264.

Lancaster, T. and Stead, L.F. (2002) Mecamylamine (a nicotine antagonist) for smoking cessation (Cochrane Review). In: *The Cochrane Library*, issue 1. Update Software, Oxford.

Mattick, R.P. and Hall, W. (1996) Are detoxification programmes effective? *The Lancet*, **347**, 97–100.

Maynard, A. and Godfrey, C. (1994) Alcohol policy – evaluating the options. *British Medical Bulletin*, **50**, 221–230.

Mayo-Smith, M.F. (1997) Pharmacological management of alcohol withdrawal. *Journal of the American Medical Association*, **278**, 144–151.

Meltzer, H., Gill, B., Pettigrew, M. and Hinds, K. (1995) *The Prevalence of Psychiatric Morbidity among Adults Living in Private Households*. HMSO, London.

Meyer, R.E. (1992) New pharmacotherapies for cocaine dependence revisited. *Archives of General Psychiatry*, **49**, 900–904.

Naranjo, C.A. and Sellers, E.M. (1986) Clinical assessment and pharmacotherapy of the alcohol withdrawal syndrome. In: *Recent Developments in Alcoholism 4* (ed. M. Galanter). Plenum Press, New York.

Newall, C.A., Anderson, L.A. and Phillipson, J.D. (1996) *Herbal Medicines: A Guide for Health-care Professionals*. Pharmaceutical Press, London, pp. 239–240.

Putzke, R., Spanagel, R., Tolle, T.R. and Zieglgansberger, W. (1996) The anti-craving drug acamprosate reduces c-fos expression in rats undergoing ethanol withdrawal. *European Journal of Pharmacology*, 317, 39–48.

Raynor, K., Kong, H., Chen, Y. *et al.* (1994) Pharmacological characterization of the cloned kappa-, delta-, and mu-opioid receptors. *Molecular Pharmacology*, 45, 330–334.

Rose, J.E., Behm, F.M., Westman, E.C. *et al.* (1994) Mecamylamine combined with nicotine skin patch facilitates smoking cessation beyond nicotine patch treatment alone. *Clinical Pharmacology and Therapeutics*, 56, 86–99.

Royal College of Psychiatrists (1986) *Alcohol: Our Favourite Drug*. Tavistock, London.

Sass, H., Soyka, M., Mann, K. and Zieglgansberger, W. (1996) Relapse prevention by acamprosate. Results from a placebo-controlled study on alcohol dependence. *Archives of General Psychiatry*, 53, 673–680.

Schuckit, M.A. (1994) The treatment of stimulant dependence. *Addiction*, 89, 1559–1563.

Schuckit, M.A., Tipp, J.E., Bergman, M. *et al.* (1997). Comparison of induced and independent major depressive disorders in 2,945 alcoholics. *American Journal of Psychiatry* 154, 948–957.

Silagy, C., Lancaster, T., Stead, L. *et al.* (2002) Nicotine replacement therapy for smoking cessation (Cochrane Review). In: *The Cochrane Library*, issue 1. Update Software, Oxford.

Srisurapanont, M. and Jarusuraisin, N. (2002) Opioid antagonists for alcohol dependence (Cochrane Review). In: *The Cochrane Library*, issue 1. Update Software, Oxford.

Whitworth, A.B., Fischer, F., Lesch, O.M. *et al.* (1996) Comparison of acamprosate and placebo in long-term treatment of alcohol dependence. *The Lancet*, 347, 1438–1442.

SELF-TEST QUESTIONS

1. Andrew is a frequent drinker of alcohol. He now needs to drink considerably more alcohol than a year ago in order to achieve the same effect. It is likely that Andrew is:
   a. changing his behaviour to overcome the effects of the alcohol
   b. becoming physiologically dependent on alcohol
   c. genetically tolerant to alcohol
   d. none of the above

2. George stopped taking amfetamine suddenly after misusing it for a considerable time. He became very ill and died, probably as a result of:
   a. substance dependence
   b. withdrawal symptoms
   c. an unrelated problem
   d. intoxication

3. The final common pathway relating to the psychopharmacology of reward is the:
   a. nigrostriatal pathway
   b. mesocortical pathway
   c. mesolimbic pathway
   d. tuberoinfundibular pathway

4. Delirium tremens refers to:
    a. the symptoms that may accompany cocaine withdrawal
    b. the symptoms associated with alcohol intoxication
    c. the symptoms that may accompany alcohol withdrawal
    d. dementia associated with alcohol misuse
5. The pharmacology of alcohol is associated with:
    a. glutamate
    b. noradrenaline (norepinephrine)
    c. serotonin
    d. GABA
6. The most important opioid receptors are the mu, delta and kappa receptors. True or false?
7. Cocaine is classified as a:
    a. stimulant
    b. hallucinogen
    c. opioid
    d. sedative
8. Benzodiazepines directly affect:
    a. dopamine levels
    b. GABA system
    c. serotonin levels
    d. noradrenaline (norepinephrine) levels
9. Ecstasy is a form of:
    a. barbiturate
    b. hallucinogen
    c. opioid
    d. stimulant
10. Flashbacks following the misuse of LSD are caused by:
    a. drug-induced altered brain structure
    b. psychological suggestion
    c. both of the above
    d. an unknown cause
11. Antabuse is a medication used with people with alcohol dependence to:
    a. stimulate vomiting when alcohol is ingested
    b. reduce craving for alcohol
    c. treat the withdrawal syndrome
    d. none of the above
12. Clonidine is used to help treat dependence on:
    a. cocaine
    b. alcohol
    c. opioids
    d. all of the above

8

THE MIND–BODY LINK

INTRODUCTION

The aim of this chapter is to introduce the reader to some of the physical conditions that can result in the person being mistakenly viewed as being mentally ill. It must also be remembered that clients can have more than one health problem, so it is useful to understand the principles of pharmacological treatment of some commonly occurring conditions, such as diabetes mellitus. A general overview of selected conditions will therefore be provided, although it is not the intention to offer a comprehensive discussion of these conditions. For further detail, the reader is advised to consult a text such as Herfindal and Gourlay, 1996 or McCance and Huether, 2001. For an introduction to general pathophysiology and pharmacology, the reader is also directed to Prosser *et al.*, 2000.

Key point ▶

> Clients may have more than one health problem. The signs of physical illness can sometimes be mistaken for those of altered mental health.

ALTERED COGNITIVE FUNCTION

Acute confusional state

As was discussed in the introductory chapter, the nerve cells are irritable. Changes in their immediate environment can alter the rate of depolarisation and thus change the way in which a person behaves, thinks or feels.

Normal cognitive function incorporates the use of reasoning, numerical calculation and appropriate language. These functions can become reversibly impaired when biochemical or physiological changes occur in the vicinity of nerve cells. Acute confusional state is a neurobehavioural syndrome (collection of signs and symptoms) that may be caused by a variety of conditions. The changes in the person's responses may be mistaken for mental illness such as psychosis or anxiety or, in older people who are more susceptible to the development of acute confusional state, the condition may be mistaken for the onset of Alzheimer's disease or another form of senile dementia.

The person in an acute confusional state may display a wide range of altered functioning of the higher centres, as shown in Table 8.1.

Alteration	Shown by
Change in consciousness Drowsiness or overanxiety	Altered arousal/wakefulness Changed attention span Altered ability to handle abstract ideas Altered insight Altered ability to recognise self
Change in perception *Illusions* – misinterpretation of sensory input *Hallucinations* – perceptions with no apparent sensory origin	Altered registering of the environment Misinterpretation of environmental sensory stimuli
Change in mood/personality Changes dependent upon original underlying personality	Altered mood and affect
Impaired problem-solving	Impaired reasoning and logic May have problems with linguistic or numerical problem-solving
Delusions – false beliefs held despite strong contradictory evidence	Irrational behaviour and communication
Delirium Agitation	Increased responsiveness to stimuli Increased neuronal activity Visual hallucinations Motor hyperactivity

Table 8.1

Alteration of cognitive functioning that may be found in people with acute confusional state.

Underlying mechanisms producing acute confusional state

Normal consciousness is usually maintained by the reticular activating system in the brain stem and thalamus and balanced functioning between the left and right hemispheres. In order for acute confusional state to develop, there is usually a malfunction of both cerebral hemispheres. Some causes of such extensive malfunction include reduced availability of the prerequisites for normal cerebral metabolism, for example hypoglycaemia (reduced blood sugar), cerebral hypoxia (reduced availability of oxygen to the brain). Acute confusional state may also be caused by acid–base or electrolyte imbalance, fever, dehydration, septicaemia (infective microorganisms in the blood), toxicity from failure of the kidneys or liver, and drug toxicity. Drug withdrawal may cause acute confusional state because of a swing in cerebral activity from under- to overactivity.

Acute confusional state can also be produced as a result of brain damage due to head injury or disease such as stroke, altered stimulation such as deprivation of sleep or sensory input, and alteration of the environment, especially in susceptible older people. Anxiety, grief and depression may also be responsible for the development of an acute confusional state, so it is important to assess the client carefully and ascertain from relatives or friends whether there is any history that may provide clues as to the underlying cause.

The effects of acute confusional state include reduced alertness, awareness and attention span, which may remain mild or progress to unconsciousness. The client may show amnesia for recent events or loss of distant recall. He or she may be unable to perform actions that require the use of logic, numerical calculations or spatial awareness, although it is important to discover before testing these what the client was good or bad at prior to the illness – some people never have been dextrous, verbally nimble or good at arithmetic! The person with acute confusional state may have rambling disorganised speech and may make errors in identifying objects that would usually be encountered every day.

It is therefore vital that patients with apparent dementia receive a proper assessment and that any physical causes are identified and remedied. For example, the older client's neural disorganisation may be miraculously improved if an underlying urinary tract or respiratory infection is treated with antibiotics. Dehydration and electrolyte imbalance is reversed by replacement of fluids. Drug toxicity should be identified from estimation of plasma levels of the medication being taken. Hepatic or renal failure can be identified by examination of blood chemistry and observation for signs such as altered urine output or jaundice. The cause of cerebral hypoxia may be a generalised respiratory infection such as bronchopneumonia, which is treated with the appropriate antibiotics and oxygen therapy.

Estimation of the blood sugar can be made using a simple finger prick test and a blood glucose meter. Usually, a hypoglycaemic person will appear pale and sweaty and may appear shaky or faint and seek food because of hunger. There may be a history of diabetes mellitus (see below) and there may be a rapid restoration to normality if glucose is

CASE STUDY 8.1   MR PATEL, A CLIENT WITH AN ACUTE CONFUSIONAL STATE

Read this case study and then attempt to answer the questions that follow.

Mr Patel is a 76-year-old retired accountant. His hobbies include golf and watching football on the television, and normally he is in good health. His wife noticed one day that he seemed not to be his usual self, he was easily irritated and was muttering to himself in an uncharacteristic fashion. This odd behaviour persisted and deteriorated over 3 days – he no longer read the newspaper and failed to follow the progress of his stocks and shares, claiming angrily that it was 'all humbug!' His family feared that he was developing Alzheimer's disease.

Mr Patel was admitted to the local hospital, where he was found to be suffering from viral pneumonia. His dehydration (due to insufficient drinking in association with being feverish) was treated and he was given oxygen and physiotherapy. As his pneumonia subsided, he resumed his perusal of the football results and the stock market and 6 weeks later was again to be seen on the golf course with his friends.

1. Why might dehydration cause the development of an acute confusional state?
2. What factors within his history would make it possible to assure his family that it would be unlikely that he had Alzheimer's disease?
3. Apart from the dehydration, what other imbalances in his central nervous system would have contributed to the confusional state?

given. The client can often be restored to healthy life and scarce mental health resources can be saved if acute confusional state is differentiated from mental illness and treated appropriately.

> Nerve cells are sensitive to changes in their local environment. Changes in the composition of extracellular fluid can alter neuronal function and produce the cognitive changes of acute confusional state. Correction of the physical disorder can restore the client to normal mental functioning.

Epilepsy

Although epilepsy may be considered by lay people to be a disease, it is produced by the effects of abnormal neurone activity, which may arise from a variety of predisposing causes. As mental health professionals frequently encounter clients who are subject to seizures, the subject of epilepsy and its pharmacological treatment will be considered in some detail here.

As has been discussed elsewhere in this book, brain functioning is regulated by the various neurotransmitters that are secreted at the synapses. Some transmitters, such as noradrenaline (norepinephrine), dopamine and serotonin, tend to stimulate neural functioning, others, such as acetylcholine and gamma-aminobutyric acid (GABA) exert a suppressive effect upon the central nervous system (CNS). If the normal biochemical balance alters in the environment surrounding the neurones, the result may be a seizure, which is an uncontrolled increase in neural activity.

Some people are more susceptible than others to the development of seizures because the readiness of their neurones to generate action potentials is enhanced, probably because of increased permeability of the neural cell membrane, enabling greater freedom of access for ions into the cell. This state is described as having a lower 'seizure threshold'. In susceptible individuals, seizures can be produced:

- as a result of biochemical imbalances such as hypoglycaemia
- following trauma, either at birth or as a result of a head injury
- in young children as a result of infection
- as a result of infection, tumours or blood vessel disease within the CNS.

Some people are genetically predisposed to seizures, which may be triggered by factors such as tiredness or physical or mental stress. Seizures may also be precipitated when stimulant drugs are taken or, in some cases, following cessation of antidepressant therapy. Other causes include respiratory alkalosis from hyperventilation (see below), certain smells or noises, premenstrual tension in women or strobe lights flashing at a certain frequency.

Key point ▶

Brain functioning is governed by neurotransmitters, some of which stimulate cerebral activity, others suppress neural functioning. An imbalance in the levels of these chemicals, or an alteration in the chemical composition of the tissue fluid in the brain may cause seizures to occur.

CASE STUDY 8.2   A CLIENT WITH EPILEPSY

Read this case study and then attempt to answer the questions that follow.

Peter, now aged 18, has minor learning difficulties and epilepsy, caused by oxygen lack to his brain at birth. He works in a carpenter's shop, and one morning, he feels one of his attacks coming on. First he smells bacon frying (it isn't), then he loses consciousness, falling to the floor with a cry, and his arms and legs become rigid. His face becomes purple, his breathing becomes laboured and his jaw is clamped tightly shut. His arms and legs then begin to convulse rhythmically for about 10 seconds, following which he becomes limp and seems to fall into a peaceful sleep.

His colleagues in the workshop have known Peter for some time, so know how to help him during such attacks.

1. What were they likely to have done for Peter while he was having this seizure?
2. When he is feeling well, Peter likes to go to the pub at lunchtime with his workmates. What must he know in order to best safeguard his health at these times?
3. If Peter's seizures seem to be increasing in frequency, what health care may be indicated?

One in 200 people in the UK have some form of epileptiform seizures. Epilepsy can be defined as recurrent episodes of uncontrolled neuronal firing, usually developing before 20 years of age. The nature of the seizures depends largely upon which area of the brain is affected, as will be discussed below.

Localised seizures

Some 'simple' seizures involve no loss of consciousness but manifest in the form of strange sensations or a characteristic smell, or the development of a particular mood or visual disturbance, psychic sensations or symptoms due to involvement of the autonomic nervous system. There may be specific motor effects, which begin in the face or hands and take the form of repetitive jerking that gradually increases in strength and speed over a period of perhaps 15 seconds, following which the movement subsides.

Jacksonian seizures begin locally and then spread to adjacent areas within the brain, so in these cases, the motor activity may begin in the fingers and then spread to the hand and forearm, finally extending over all of one side of the body before ceasing spontaneously. Sensory seizures may involve feelings of numbness, burning or tingling, paraesthesia ('pins and needles') or sensations of crawling or movements of body parts. Focal seizures usually involve local neurones in the cerebral cortex on one side of the brain only. **Temporal lobe seizures** may be associated with **automatism** which is the ability to interact with the environment even though movements may be inappropriate and the individual is not fully aware of his/her actions. There may be characteristic sensations of taste, sound or smell, accompanied by repetitive behaviour such as lip-smacking, facial grimacing or repetitive rubbing or plucking actions. Such seizures tend to last for less than 5 minutes and are followed by a short period of confusion.

◄ *Key point*

> Localised seizures involve no overall loss of consciousness, but the person may experience altered sensations, or abnormal movements may be noticeable for a short period of time.

Generalised seizures

These involve both hemispheres of the brain and often originate from a source deep within the cerebral tissue. Prior to the development of the seizure, the individual may experience prodromal sensations, which may provide a warning 'aura' heralding the onset of an attack. Generalised seizures involve widespread neuronal discharges and loss of normal consciousness. **Absence seizures**, otherwise known as **petit mal attacks**, originate from multiple areas of the brain and develop in children older than 4 years of age. A brief loss of contact with the immediate environment occurs: the child stops activity and appears vacant for 5–10 seconds, although s/he will respond if spoken to. The child either eventually 'grows out of' the condition or develops major seizures in adulthood.

Atonic seizures, otherwise known as **'drop attacks'** or **akinetic seizures** are multifocal seizures that result in a sudden loss of tone in the postural muscles and subsequent inability to maintain the position in space.

Myoclonic seizures are characterised by momentary loss of consciousness associated with vigorous jerking of one or more limbs or the entire body. Following the attack, there is a short period of **postictal** (post-seizure) confusion. Such attacks may occur in clusters. **Clonic seizures** are characterised by alternating episodes of rigidity and relaxation of major muscle groups. The convulsions decline in strength as the attack subsides.

In **tonic–clonic seizures**, previously known as grand mal epilepsy, the fit has a characteristic series of phases. The seizure may be heralded by an aura during which the individual has feelings of irritability or specific sensory experiences. Many tonic–clonic seizures, however, occur without warning. There is a loss of consciousness and the person falls to the ground, usually with the limbs extended and the muscles rigid. The jaw muscles are in spasm and breathing is affected. The individual may be cyanosed with the pupils dilated and unresponsive to light. Although this stage of the seizure may be mistaken for a cardiorespiratory arrest, it is unwise to try to clear the airway of someone in a tonic–clonic seizure as the strength of contraction of the jaw muscle is not easily overcome, fingers entering the mouth may be badly bitten and the use of instruments will only cause damage to the sufferer's teeth. During this phase of the seizure, which lasts between 15 seconds and 1 minute, the bladder or bowel may be involuntarily voided.

The tonic phase is succeeded by the clonic phase, during which regular violent generalised muscle contractions take place. Respirations resume and hyperventilation occurs, and eye rolling, facial contortion and salivation are evident. The pulse is rapid and profuse sweating is evident. Usually, within about 30 seconds, the clonic contractions subside and the person becomes limp, the breathing becomes quieter and, although unconsciousness remains, the pupils begin to react to light. As recovery proceeds, consciousness is regained but the person is dazed and confused, has no memory of the convulsion and may complain of muscle pain and fatigue. The principles of care for someone undergoing a generalised convulsion are shown in Table 8.2.

Table 8.2 Principles of care for a person undergoing a tonic–clonic convulsion.	**Phase**	**Action**
	Prodromal stage	Individual may learn to recognise prodromal signs and seek a safe place before consciousness is lost
	Tonic stage	If possible, remove any hazards form the person's vicinity. Do not try to force the mouth open or otherwise interfere unnecessarily. Stage usually lasts less than 1 minute. If possible, provide privacy.
	Clonic stage	As for tonic stage. Usually subsides within 30 seconds, although both tonic and clonic states may seem to last longer as they can be disturbing to observe
	Postictal stage	Help patient to reorientate, restore normal appearance and rest after attack

During the postictal phase there may be a time when, although conscious, the individual's behaviour has not yet returned to normal and there is diminished responsibility for personal actions. The tonic–clonic attacks may occur during sleep or waking hours and may recur unpredictably at intervals ranging from hours to years later.

In a few cases, the tonic–clonic episode may not subside and the individual enters a state of status epilepticus in which successive convulsive episodes occur. This is a medical emergency as the constant violent muscular contractions may cause bodily damage and the heat generated from the constant muscular activity causes the body temperature to rise. If the resultant high fever is not treated, death may occur as a result either of the denaturing of body proteins because of the abnormal body heat or of hypoxia from the respiratory disorganisation caused by the constant convulsions. Treatment is to transfer the patient to a general hospital with intensive care facilities and give anticonvulsants, possibly to paralyse the muscle temporarily and institute artificial ventilation of the lungs in addition to reducing the body temperature to normal limits.

Patients who have a history of major convulsions are precluded from driving or riding motorcycles, usually until they have been free from attacks for a period of 2 years, with or without medication. Some forms of major seizure are associated, either by cause or effect, with learning difficulties and in some cases there are personality disorders. However, epilepsy is a common phenomenon with an incidence equalling that of diabetes mellitus (see below). It is important to realise that it occurs in all sections of society, including some gifted and influential people such as Julius Caesar.

Epilepsy is diagnosed by the presence of characteristic 'spike and wave' electroencephalogram complexes, which may be evoked by stimuli during the investigation. The patient's history and brain scans are used to exclude other possible causes of convulsive seizures.

Waveform prior
to seizure

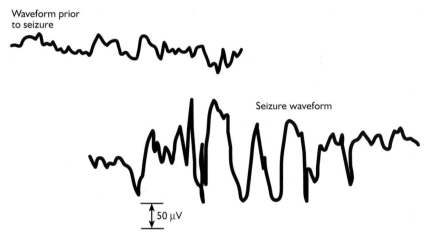

Seizure waveform

50 μV

In a major fit, the seizure waveform is seen
simultaneously across a large number of
electrodes indicating different regions of the brain

Figure 8.1

The electroencephalogram complex
diagnostic of epilepsy

◄ **Key point**

Epileptic seizures take many different forms. Tonic–clonic seizures involve loss of consciousness and usually follow a pattern of stages, during which the major aim of care is to prevent the person from suffering physical harm and to protect their privacy and dignity.

Pharmacological treatment of convulsive seizures

The aim of treatment is to reduce the neural over-reactivity and thus protect the person against further seizures. Doses need careful regulation to achieve optimal control of the convulsive seizures. In the case of pregnant women who have seizures, there are inherent problems related to managing the pregnancy and the medication: the medication may cause fetal abnormalities but cessation of anticonvulsant medication can provoke seizures, which are also dangerous for the fetus.

Carbamazepine is given to control tonic–clonic and partial seizures. 100–200 mg twice daily may be given, with the dose being gradually adjusted. Doses of more than 1200 mg daily are usually avoided. The medication is presented in chewable, orange-flavoured tablets as well as the standard pressed tablet format. Plasma levels may be monitored as carbamazepine is erratically absorbed from the gastrointestinal tract and is removed from the body by hepatic metabolism. Adverse effects include dizziness, drowsiness, nausea and anorexia and carbamazepine can also produce depression, irritability and lapses in concentration and short-term memory. Rashes can occur and erythrocyte and white cell counts may be monitored as aplastic anaemia can occur on rare occasions. Clients and their families should be advised to report fevers, sore throat, rashes, mouth ulcers or unexplained bruising.

Carbamazepine is chemically related to the tricyclic antidepressant imipramine and is useful as treatment for tonic–clonic and partial seizures. It is thought to reduce excessive neuronal firing by influencing the sodium channels along the nerve cell membrane, thus reducing the generation of action potentials and transmission across synapses. Carbamazepine influences the activity of some liver enzymes and for this reason this medication may reduce the effectiveness of hormones used as oral contraceptives. Because it also slows the electrical conduction in the heart, carbamazepine should be avoided if possible in patients with disturbances of cardiac rhythm. Latent psychoses and in elderly clients, agitation and confusion, may occur, particularly when high doses of the drug are used.

A range of drug interactions occur as carbamazepine increases the metabolism in the liver of drugs such as clobazam, clonazepam, primidone, valproic acid, alprazolam, haloperidol, imipramine and methadone and may increase or decrease the effectiveness of phenytoin (see below). Overdosage of carbamazepine alters the functioning of the CNS and the cardiorespiratory systems. Depression, drowsiness, agitation confusion and coma may occur, also, paradoxically, convulsions. Respiratory depression and tachycardia, possibly with irregular pulse and hyper- or hypotension, may occur.

Phenytoin acts as an anticonvulsant by blocking sodium and calcium conductance across the nerve cell membrane. It is available as a suspension, capsules or tablets. This preparation is useful for the treatment of partial fits and the control of tonic–clonic seizures. A dose of 300 mg daily is given as a starting dose and the amount is gradually adjusted subsequently to avoid saturation of hepatic enzymes. Different individuals metabolise phenytoin differently, so it is difficult to predict the effect a given dosage will have. Changes of dosage need to be carried out gradually and ideally the client is prescribed the lowest dose that effectively controls seizures. In most adults 200–500 mg daily in single or divided doses will be effective. Particular care is needed with the dosage for older clients.

Adverse effects include ataxia, diplopia (double vision) dizziness, drowsiness and the development of involuntary movements. If medication with phenytoin is suddenly stopped, there is a risk of provoking status epilepticus. A sudden large intake of alcohol may produce increased plasma levels of phenytoin, and the levels may diminish in clients who are chronic alcohol abusers. In some clients, the combination of phenytoin with tricyclic antidepressants or phenothiazines may cause seizures to occur. Overdose of phenytoin produces unresponsive pupils, coma and hypotension, also respiratory depression and cessation of breathing. An overdose of 2–5 g may be lethal in adults.

Valproic acid and **sodium valproate** are used to control partial and generalised seizures respectively. Valproate is also useful for absence seizures. It is thought to act as an agonist of GABA. A starting dose of 125–300 mg three times daily is usually prescribed for adults and then increased. The effective dose is usually 750–1300 mg daily given in three or four divided doses. It is available as enteric-coated capsules, which should be swallowed whole.

Valproate is usually well tolerated, the most common adverse effects being gastrointestinal symptoms, although it can cause weight gain and hair loss. When prescribed in combination with other anticonvulsant agents, the effective dose becomes unpredictable and may need to be adjusted upwards or downwards to keep seizures under control. Liver function may be impaired as a result of treatment with valproate so episodes of nausea, fat intolerance or jaundice should be reported. Some people become sedated or aggressive or develop hyperactivity tremor or ataxia when treated with this group of anticonvulsants. In common with other anticonvulsants, treatment during pregnancy is problematic, but it is safe for use by breast feeding mothers. Minor overdosage is not particularly dangerous; respiratory and nervous system depression are dangers in large overdoses.

Ethosuximide is used for absence seizures in young children, or for absence seizures in combination with tonic–clonic convulsions. It is thought to alter calcium movement in the thalamus and possibly to deplete excitatory neurotransmitters within the CNS. Seizures seem to be reduced by depression of activity in the motor cortex of the brain and increase of the threshold for seizures in the CNS. It is available as syrup and capsules. For adults and children over 6 years of age, the dose is adjusted upwards from a starting dose of 500 mg daily until control of the seizures is achieved.

Fetal abnormality may occur if treatment is needed during pregnancy and the drug is secreted in breast milk, so it is not suitable for use by lactating mothers. At the onset of treatment, apathy, drowsiness, depression or slight euphoria may occur, also headaches, dizziness and ataxia. Such adverse reactions may resolve spontaneously. Care is needed for clients with liver or kidney dysfunction, and the agent will interact if prescribed in combination with other anticonvulsant drugs. Ethosuximide can cause weight loss, skin rashes, gum enlargement and gastrointestinal disturbances. Large overdoses may produce coma and respiratory depression.

Gabapentin is a derivative of GABA. It is used in the treatment of partial and generalised tonic–clonic seizures and is available as 100 mg, 300 mg and 400 mg capsules. Usually, doses of 900–1200 mg daily are needed to control seizures, and such doses can be built up fairly quickly. Discontinuation or addition of other anticonvulsant therapy is usually undertaken gradually, although this product is relatively unreactive with other anticonvulsants. In addition, gabapentin can be taken with oral contraceptive preparations as it does not alter the bioavailability of these hormones.

The preparation has not been identified as safe for use during pregnancy or lactation. In older clients, diminishing renal function may mean that a reduced dose is needed. Generally, gabapentin has been found to be relatively free of dangerous adverse effects but sleepiness, ataxia, double vision, headache nausea and vomiting may occur. Drowsiness appears to be the main problem when significant overdosage occurs.

Lamotrigine works by inhibiting the voltage-dependent sodium channels in the neuronal cell wall and producing a decrease in the excitatory neurotransmitters aspartate and glutamate. It is available in tablet form and is used for simple or complex partial seizures and tonic–clonic seizures. For adults and children over 12 years, 25 mg is taken once a day for 2 weeks, followed by 50 mg once a day for the same period of time. The dose is then increased by 50–100 mg every 1–2 weeks until seizures are controlled.

The dose needs to be carefully regulated if the client is receiving other enzyme-inducing antiepileptic medication, such as phenytoin, carbamazepine, phenobarbital and primidone, as hepatic enzymes can either be induced or inhibited, thus making therapy unpredictable. Skin reactions, which may occasionally be serious, may develop in association with treatment with lamotrigine and headache, nausea, dizziness, visual disturbances and ataxia may occur. Generally, the effects of overdosage are not serious.

Phenobarbital (phenobarbitone) was first used as treatment in 1912. The agent is thought to increase the seizure threshold by acting as a GABA agonist or as an antagonist of the excitatory neurotransmitter glutamate. It tends to cause sedation. Its use has now largely been super-seded by other anticonvulsant agents.

Primidone works in a similar manner to phenobarbital as it is metabolised to phenobarbital. Major depression of the CNS is produced by treatment. Its use is indicated for clients with major tonic–clonic convulsions, temporal lobe epilepsy and for some focal and Jacksonian fits. The dose is gradually augmented and adults may require 1.5 g per day in divided doses to control seizures. It can be used in combination with other anticonvulsants, although the problem of interaction with hepatic enzymes alters the predictability of treatment. Rapid cessation of primidone may cause status epilepticus. Tolerance or dependence may occur and withdrawal reactions may develop if the medication is ceased abruptly.

Primidone enhances the effect of alcohol and reduces the effectiveness of oral contraceptives. Congenital abnormalities may occur if the drug is taken during pregnancy and breastfed babies may become sedated by the mother's medication. Drowsiness, skin rashes, ataxia, headaches, nausea and vomiting and visual disturbances may occur. Overdosage causes depression of the CNS.

> The dose of medication used for the treatment of epileptic seizures must be carefully titrated against the client's symptoms. Many anticonvulsants influence the functioning of liver enzymes, which may cause difficulties when the client needs also to be treated with a range of other drugs for conditions other than epilepsy.

◄ *Key point*

If a client enters **status epilepticus**, pharmacological control of the seizures must be achieved urgently. In such cases, anticonvulsant therapy must be given intravenously, using drugs such as diazepam, phenobarbital or phenytoin. Other agents that may be used intravenously include **clonazepam, lorazepam** or **clomethiazole** (chlormethiazole). If the seizures cannot be controlled by other means, the client may require a general anaesthetic and neuromuscular blockade to achieve paralysis until the convulsions cease. Such treatment would require transfer to a general hospital with intensive care facilities as artificial ventilation would be required to prevent asphyxia due to paralysis of the respiratory muscles.

PHYSICAL DISORDERS ORIGINATING FROM ALTERED AROUSAL

Stress-related disorders

The physiological adaptations to short- and long-term stress are set out in Chapter 2. In summary, psychological stress causes a series of neural and endocrine responses that serve to maintain the individual in a dynamic state of readiness to deal with challenge. The study of stress has led to the development of the science of psychoneuroimmunology and the proposition that disease has multiple causation. The nervous and endocrine systems are closely interlinked at the level of the hypothalamus and pituitary and also in the adrenal gland, where the medulla is activated by nerve stimuli to release adrenaline (epinephrine) and noradrenaline (norepinephrine) as a result of stimulation by nerve endings. The adrenal cortex is stimulated to release corticosteroids by adrenocorticotrophic hormone (ACTH). A prolonged unresolved stress response has been noted to be linked with altered adrenocortical functioning and to be associated with pathological changes.

A number of conditions are now thought to be caused at least in part by a maladaptive stress response. These include coronary artery disease, hypertension, stroke and alterations to the cardiac rhythm such as paroxysmal tachycardia (rapid heart rate) and atrial fibrillation. Bronchial asthma and hyperventilation syndrome (see below) may alter the functioning of the respiratory system. Within the alimentary tract, ulceration of the lining of the stomach or duodenum may occur, or there may be alterations to the normal bowel motility resulting in diarrhoea, irritable bowel syndrome, nausea and vomiting, or inflammatory bowel disease, which may cause pain, diarrhoea and impaired absorption of nutrients. Increased muscle tension may result in tension headaches or backache. Altered immune responses can be associated with the development of rheumatoid arthritis.

The immune system itself may diminish in competence predisposing to infection, delayed healing or the development of malignant tumours. The latter develop if lymphocytes (the white cells that are able to detect and destroy abnormal tissue) become less vigilant and fail to recognise markers on newly formed cells that indicate that the cell's DNA has mutated. Conversely, the immune system may become overactive and there may be overproduction of antibodies and activation of the white cells against normal tissue.

Chronic maladaptive stress may result in sexual dysfunction or infertility. The stress response has also been implicated in the development of diabetes mellitus. Changes within the CNS can result in altered sleep patterns (see Chapter 2), eating disorders, lethargy and tiredness, depression or 'driven' Type A behaviour.

Key point ▶

> As well as being an unpleasant experience for the sufferer, long-term psychological stress is associated with a range of physical disorders.

Hyperventilation syndrome

The term 'hyperventilation' is used to describe a state in which the respiratory effort made by the individual is in excess of that needed to meet the metabolic needs. Normally, the rate of breathing is controlled by the respiratory centre in the medulla oblongata in response to the activity of chemoreceptors, which relay neural stimuli to alter breathing according to the levels of carbon dioxide and pH in the blood and cerebrospinal fluid. Oxygen lack in blood also stimulates respiration, although, in health and normal atmosphere at sea level, this mechanism is seldom activated.

When a person has hyperventilation syndrome, a range of stimuli can invoke inappropriate respiratory effort. Causes that include breath-holding, accumulation of lactic acid and emotional stress stimulate the sufferer to breathe at an inappropriate rate and depth. The result is that excessive loss of carbon dioxide from the blood occurs, which makes the person feel lightheaded and may cause tetany, in which there is spasm of the muscles of the hands and feet, and a tingling sensation around the mouth. This is due to calcium shifts in the blood, which

CASE STUDY 8.3   JOAN, A CLIENT WITH HYPERVENTILATION SYNDROME

Read this case study and then attempt to answer the questions that follow.

Joan is a naturally anxious person. Recently she has become preoccupied with her breathing, which she feels to be inadequate – she has to take occasional extra deep breaths on a regular basis and if she gets upset she finds that her breathing 'runs away from her', in that she feels she can't keep up with her need for air and so breathes faster and faster. As she does so, she feels dizzy and lightheaded, which leads her to conclude that she isn't getting enough air, so a vicious circle ensues and she breathes harder and faster, feels even more lightheaded and gets a sense of numbness around the mouth and a feeling of crushing heaviness in her chest.

1. How would you explain to Joan how she might control her symptoms?
2. Why would it be better for her health in the long run if she could break free of this pattern of overbreathing?
3. Joan is referred for a course of cognitive behavioural therapy. What medication might be useful as an adjunct to help her to overcome this problem?

---

occur in an attempt to correct the alkalosis caused by the hyperventilation. The strange feelings may cause the person to panic and further hyperventilate, thus creating a vicious circle. Chronic hyperventilation syndrome can cause further frightening symptoms such as chest pain due to coronary artery spasm and alterations to the blood pressure. Hyperventilation sufficient to cause respiratory alkalosis also causes vasoconstriction of the cerebral blood vessels.

People with psychogenic hyperventilation often complain of feeling breathless at rest and report frequent feelings of needing to sigh. It is often possible to demonstrate to the patient that rebreathing into a paper bag to increase the carbon dioxide levels and restore the pH, will bring the symptoms under control. For some, beta-adrenergic-blocking drugs such as propranolol are helpful to control feelings of anxiety and tachyarrhythmias (rapid irregular pulse rates) that may arise. Anxiety management courses or exercise programmes are also helpful for some sufferers.

◀ **Key point**

> Hyperventilation syndrome occurs when the client makes sustained respiratory effort that is in excess of metabolic needs. Hyperventilation may cause disturbing symptoms and, if it remains uncontrolled, constriction of blood vessels within the brain or myocardium may cause symptoms and impaired function due to reduced oxygen delivery to these organs.

OTHER DISORDERS OF PARTICULAR INTEREST TO MENTAL HEALTH PROFESSIONALS

The conditions considered in the remainder of this chapter are presented in overview. It is important to be aware of these conditions, which may mistakenly be thought to be a presentation of mental illness. Detailed discussion of medication used for these conditions can be found in texts concerned with general pathophysiology and pharmacology.

DISORDERS OF THE ENDOCRINE SYSTEM

Disorders of the thyroid gland

The thyroid acts under the control of the hypothalamus and pituitary gland to regulate the rate of cellular metabolism by its secretion of thyroxine (T_4) and triiodothyronine (T_3). The thyroid gland is located in the neck, anterior to the larynx, and some cases of thyroid disorder involve a swelling of the gland, which results in enlargement of the neck, so the client may complain that collars or necklaces have become too tight. Disorders of the thyroid may therefore produce in the client an overall state of over- or underactivity. The client needs estimation of plasma thyroid hormone levels to help to differentiate symptoms due to endocrine abnormalities from those due to mental illness.

As a general rule, people with thyroid disorders gradually change in appearance and activity over a period of time (Figure 8.2). They and their close associates may not notice any difference and it may only be when they meet someone who has not seen them for a period of months or years that a change is noticed.

Key point ▶

> Endocrine disorders tend to develop slowly. Although alteration to the client's appearance may result, this is usually more noticeable to those who meet them after a period of time has elapsed.

Thyrotoxicosis (overactivity of the thyroid gland) produces an increased metabolic rate. There are various causes of this condition: sometimes it is the result of altered immunity, which results in the production of an antibody that binds to thyroid cells and acts as a thyroid-stimulating substance. This in turn causes the thyroid to secrete more T_3 and T_4, which then increase the metabolic rate. The person with hyperthyroidism may present with a selection or all of the following symptoms. Restlessness, overactivity and anxiety are common, as is weight loss, tachycardia (increased heart rate), tremor, heat intolerance, sweating and diarrhoea. People with severe symptoms may have physical changes such as thinning of the hair and exophthalmos – bulging of the eyes, which is due to the accumulation of a fatty deposit within the orbit. In extreme cases, thyrotoxicosis may be associated with the development of euphoric or psychotic states.

Clearly, symptoms of an overactive thyroid need to be differentiated from those of generalised anxiety states because the treatment differs in some important respects. It should be remembered that anxiety may have an underlying cause of thyroid overactivity, also that a patient with an overactive thyroid may well develop anxiety syndromes.

Beta-adrenergic blockers are used to treat anxiety and also other symptoms of thyroid overactivity such as tachycardia and overactivity. However, other specific antithyroid drugs such as **carbimazole** and **propylthiouracil** may be prescribed to block the thyroid's use of iodine to make T_3 and T_4 and thus return the metabolic rate to normal levels.

Overactivity of the thyroid gland may cause the individual to become anxious and hyperactive as well as producing a range of physiological changes consistent with an increased metabolic rate.

◀ *Key point*

We have seen how overactivity of the thyroid gland is associated with states that can be confused with anxiety disorders. The thyroid may begin to fail because of reduced stimulus from the pituitary or the hypothalamus as a result of overly effective treatment of hyperthyroidism, or because of auto immune destruction of thyroid tissue. When the thyroid becomes underactive, the client becomes slower and less responsive and this state may be confused with depressive states or the onset of dementia. People with **myxoedema** (thyroid underactivity) tend to gain weight, become more drowsy and feel the cold. Abnormal mucopolysaccharides and proteins are deposited in the skin and connective tissue; this attracts water through osmosis, causing oedema, which is particularly noticeable around the eyes and in the hands and feet, so rings and shoes may no longer fit. The person with an underactive thyroid may become mentally slower and may have thinning of the hair, voice changes such as hoarseness due to the myxoedemic deposits around the larynx, and enlargement of the tongue, which will change the facial appearance over a period of time. Constipation, irregularity or cessation of menstruation and reduced muscle strength may all contribute to a mistaken conclusion that premature ageing has occurred. It is not unheard of for such a person to be admitted to a long-stay facility and then to make a miraculous recovery when the thyroid disorder is finally identified and treated!

Thyroid underactivity is confirmed by low levels of T_3 and T_4 in the plasma and the treatment is by life-long replacement of the deficient thyroid hormone. Thyroxine is usually given but triiodothyronine may be used in the rapid treatment of acute, severe hypothyroid states.

Underactivity of the thyroid may produce signs and symptoms which may be confused with those of clinical depression or premature ageing.

◀ *Key point*

Figure 8.2

Common changes in appearance accompanying alteration in thyroid function.

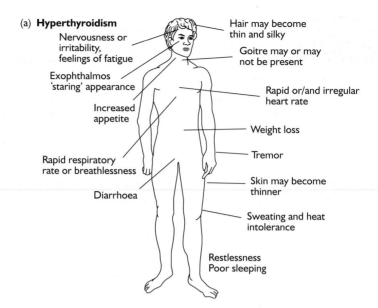

(a) **Hyperthyroidism**

Nervousness or irritability, feelings of fatigue

Exophthalmos 'staring' appearance

Increased appetite

Rapid respiratory rate or breathlessness

Diarrhoea

Hair may become thin and silky

Goitre may or may not be present

Rapid or/and irregular heart rate

Weight loss

Tremor

Skin may become thinner

Sweating and heat intolerance

Restlessness Poor sleeping

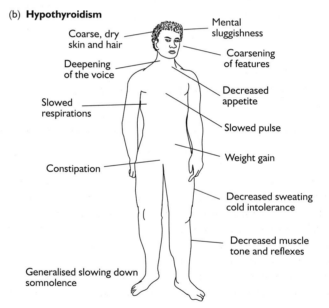

(b) **Hypothyroidism**

Coarse, dry skin and hair

Deepening of the voice

Slowed respirations

Constipation

Generalised slowing down somnolence

Mental sluggishness

Coarsening of features

Decreased appetite

Slowed pulse

Weight gain

Decreased sweating cold intolerance

Decreased muscle tone and reflexes

Diabetes mellitus

Diabetes mellitus is sufficiently prevalent in the population to coexist with mental illness in some clients, so an awareness of the principles of care may be helpful.

Glucose homeostasis

Glucose is an energy fuel that is used for cerebral metabolism. The cells of CNS are always able to extract glucose from the bloodstream in

| CASE STUDY 8.4 | HALMA AND MISS SPINKS, TWO WOMEN WITH THYROID DISORDERS MIMICKING MENTAL ILLNESS |

Read this case study and then attempt to answer the questions that follow.

Halma went to see her family doctor asking for a prescription to help her contain her anxious feelings. She was complaining of 'feeling jittery', having sweaty palms, trembling fingers and a racing pulse. She had been losing weight over the past 4 months, although she was, in her own words, 'eating like a horse'. She was glad it was now winter, as she found heat intolerable, despite having originally been born and brought up in a hot country. Her doctor thought she might have a thyroid disorder, so sent a blood sample for thyroid function tests.

1. From her symptoms, is Halma likely to have an overactive or underactive thyroid gland?
2. Explain why any pre-existing tendency towards anxiety would be made worse by this thyroid disorder
3. What are the risks of untreated hyperthyroidism?

Miss Marjorie Spinks is a lady of 76 who lives alone in a detached house. She dreads the winter because she has found, as the years go by, that she really cannot bear the cold – she tends to stay in bed a lot in winter or to crouch over the electric fire. Her winter coat and other warm clothes no longer fit, because of a sustained weight gain. She feels lethargic and is finally persuaded by her neighbour to accept a visit from her family practice. When the family doctor sees her, she finds Miss Spinks to be an overweight, passive lady who feels cold and complains of weight gain and constipation. She has scorch marks on the front of her lower legs. The doctor sends Miss Spinks to hospital for assessment and stabilisation of her thyroid condition.

4. Is Miss Spinks' thyroid likely to be over- or underactive?
5. If she had continued untreated, what risks would there have been to her health?
6. Why might such clients sometimes be erroneously considered to be depressed or suffering from symptoms of early dementia?

order to synthesise adenosine triphosphate to fuel cerebral functioning. When glucose is present in the plasma in abundant supply, it is made available for use by all cells through the secretion of **insulin** by the beta cells of the islets of Langerhans in the pancreas. Insulin acts as a carrier protein that enables glucose to enter all cells. During times of fasting, such as a night's sleep, a limited amount of glucose is made available by release from stores in the liver. This occurs when the hormone glucagon is secreted from alpha cells, also in the Isles of Langerhans in the pancreas.

Normally, therefore, the brain has constant access to its major energy fuel, glucose. Other body cells have access to this energy compound on a rationing basis, the hormone controlling the 'rationing' being insulin and the hormone unlocking emergency stores at times when the brain is at risk of being deprived of glucose being glucagon. Thus, glucagon is the hormone that raises the blood glucose level and insulin reduces it, the aim at all times being to maintain the vital cerebral functioning by ensuring a priority supply of glucose to the brain and CNS.

Should the emergency supply of glucose, stored in the form of glycogen, become depleted, most organs of the body except the brain are able to use an alternative energy compound in the form of fatty acids obtained from breakdown of the fat stores in the adipose tissue. Unfortunately, if liberated in large amounts, the ketoacids that are the end product of fatty acid metabolism produce a toxic depressive effect upon neural functioning. So, if the availability of glucose for energy is compromised, this produces effects upon cerebral functioning: the person with **hypoglycaemia** (low blood glucose) is likely to feel anxious, shaky and sweaty and to look pale. If the hypoglycaemia is not rectified by the ingestion of some readily absorbed glucose, fainting, convulsions, coma and ultimately death will occur. The person who has excessive ketoacids in the bloodstream will feel unwell and become confused and drowsy. Figure 8.3 summarises the mechanisms of glucose homeostasis.

Figure 8.3

Glucose homeostasis

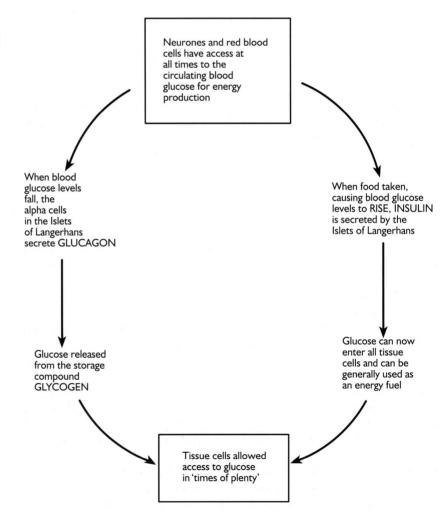

> The CNS uses glucose as its main energy source. When glucose levels in the blood are high, insulin is secreted and glucose is then made generally available for widespread cell metabolism. When blood glucose levels are low, glycogen causes glucose to be released from storage for metabolism within the CNS.

Diabetes mellitus is a condition that results in altered availability of glucose because of impaired production or effectiveness of insulin. The name comes from the Greek for 'sweetness running through'. The 'running' refers to the increased fluid intake and urine output, which the ancient Greek physicians noticed. In the absence of reagents used for testing the chemical constituents of urine, the physicians used to taste urine, and found that the urine of diabetic patients tasted 'like honey' because of the abnormal presence of glucose (glycosuria)! Glycosuria occurs for many reasons. Normally the kidneys return all glucose from the urinary filtrate to the bloodstream by active transport. However, if there is an overload of glucose in the bloodstream beyond the renal threshold, there are insufficient chemical transport mechanisms to return all of the glucose and some remains within the urine. The renal threshold can become altered in pregnancy and in patients taking corticosteroids or other drugs, thus producing glycosuria. However, diabetes mellitus constitutes a separate series of disorders in which either insufficient insulin is produced or ineffective insulin fails to enable carriage of glucose into cells. The brain continues to get its vital supplies, but the other tissues of the body are deprived and are obliged to use alternative sources of energy while the unused glucose accumulates in the plasma. The result is a high blood sugar and glycosuria.

Weight loss, hunger and fatigue occur because of the long-term deprivation of the energy compound to the cells. Infections occur because the excessive glucose is used as a nutritive medium by microorganisms. The patient's CNS may be affected by ketoacidosis or by osmotic shifts due to the effect of the glucose and ketoacids in the bloodstream, which draw water from the cerebral tissue and thus cause dehydration of the CNS. In such unresolved cases, drowsiness, convulsions, coma and death would be the final outcome.

Detailed management of the patient with uncontrolled diabetes mellitus is not the concern of the mental health worker but it is important to be aware of the outcome of undetected or poorly managed diabetes mellitus. It may be necessary to encourage the client to monitor his/her own blood sugar and to understand that, in such clients, alterations in arousal or cognitive function may have a metabolic, rather than a psychiatric cause.

Clients with **type 1 diabetes** have a form of the condition in which the islet cells of the pancreas have failed to secrete sufficient insulin; these people must take insulin replacement therapy for life. Insulin is destroyed by first-pass metabolism, so the medication must be taken as an injection to avoid the destruction that would otherwise occur in the alimentary tract. Such clients may display the signs of hypogly-caemia (see above) if excessive insulin is taken, and this must be corrected with glucose to maintain cerebral function and prevent permanent damage.

Other clients display some of the signs of diabetes mellitus, often later in life, but their symptoms can be controlled by oral medication. This is because they have **type 2 diabetes**: insulin is being produced but medication is needed to strengthen the cell receptors' response to it or to enhance intracellular mechanisms that enable usage of the glucose in the mitochondria. Products such as **chlorpropamide**, **tolbutamide**, **glibenclamide** and **gliclazide** are examples of oral hypoglycaemic agents that may be used by clients with type 2 diabetes. Although this form is also called non-insulin-dependent diabetes mellitus (abbreviated to NIDDM), this is a somewhat confusing term, as insulin is sometimes needed to restore glycaemic control in such clients.

In some milder cases, the diabetes can be controlled purely by dietary control of simple carbohydrates; again, this would be primarily the responsibility of other health professionals but the client may need encouragement to comply with necessary modifications to the lifestyle. It is important to be aware that an insulin-using client who is suicidal has a very potent means of irreversible self harm at his/her disposal.

For a more comprehensive discussion of this complex condition, the reader is advised to consult a textbook of general pathophysiology such as McCance and Huether, 2001.

Key point ▶

> In diabetes mellitus, there is either a failure of insulin production, or faulty response to insulin by the cells. The result is that glucose cannot be taken into the cells for energy creation, so it remains in the bloodstream in increased amounts, some spilling over into the urine where its presence can be identified during routine urinalysis.

Cushing's disease

This condition is mentioned briefly here as it sometimes causes emotional lability or psychosis that could result in referral for mental health care. Cushing's disease results from overactivity of the adrenal cortex and, therefore, excessive production of cortisol. A similar picture occurs in Cushing's syndrome, which occurs in patients who have needed to take large doses of corticosteroids. The effects include: weight gain, particularly in the trunk; acne; hypertension; development of facial hair in females; reduced immune response; impaired healing; and glycosuria. The client requires investigation and treatment of the underlying cause, in which case the mental disorder should resolve.

ORGANIC BRAIN DISEASE

As has been discussed in the context of examples such as diabetes mellitus and acute confusional state, marked neurophysiological malfunctioning can result from a purely physical cause. Below, a brief summary is given of some other physical causes of abnormal mental functioning. For a more detailed insight than is possible here, the reader is once again referred to a comprehensive pathophysiology text.

Space-occupying lesions within the central nervous system

We have seen that chemical changes within the brain are likely to alter neural functioning, which is why the blood–brain barrier has developed as a protection. Sometimes, altered behaviour or mood provide an early sign that some abnormal structure is causing pressure within the cranial cavity. This could be caused by cerebral tumours, bleeds due to trauma or blood vessel disease, or inflammation surrounding an infarction (cell death) of cerebral tissue due to an interruption of normal blood supply, such as occurs in cases of cerebral thrombosis.

The brain can be likened to a blancmange that is supported within a bone box. The delicate nature of the neural tissue makes the CNS vulnerable to disruption due to displacement if some alteration to the normal anatomy occurs. Of course, this is why the 'bone box' of the cranium exists, but its very rigidity means that, should for some reason swelling of the brain occur, there is very little free space to accommodate the resultant change in the brain's volume. In fact, the only break in the uniform rigidity of the cranium is at the foramen magnum, the aperture that allows the spinal cord to leave the cranium. Unfortunately, the cranial nerves controlling activation of the autonomic functions such as maintenance of the heart rate and breathing also emerge from the foramen magnum. If raised intracranial pressure forces the brain downwards towards this aperture, then the cranial nerves will be at risk of compression, which will stop the heart and breathing and kill the patient.

Generally, a sudden unexplained alteration in consciousness in an otherwise well person, particularly associated with a history of headache, nausea and vomiting or previous head injury, all of which may indicate raised intracranial pressure, needs physical investigation as a matter of some urgency. Unrelieved brain swelling will result in cardiorespiratory collapse and subsequent death, so transfer to a specialist neurosurgical unit may be needed in some cases.

Altered mental functioning may sometimes be the result of conditions that cause compression of the brain because of injury or disease. It is important that these potentially life-threatening states are recognised as being of physical, rather than mental, origin and receive the appropriate treatment.

SUMMARY

The mind and the body are closely linked and signs of physical ill-health sometimes resemble those of mental illness. It is important that the nature of the condition is properly understood so that the appropriate treatment is given to the client. Mentally ill clients may become physically ill as well; this also has to be recognised and dealt with accordingly. Systemic biochemical abnormalities may produce disorders of cognition or seizures due to changes in the composition of the cerebral extracellular fluid. Psychological stress may generate physical as well as mental ill-health. Certain endocrinological disorders or cerebral compression may caused altered behaviour that may be misinterpreted as the effects of a mental illness or inappropriate use of alcohol or drugs. A failure to identify these problems may have serious repercussions for the client's future health.

REFERENCES AND FURTHER READING

Herfindal, E.T. and Gourlay, D.R. (1996) *Textbook of Therapeutics and Disease Management*. Williams & Wilkins, Baltimore, MD.

McCance, K.L. and Huether, S.E. (2001) *Pathophysiology: The Biological Basis for Disease in Adults and Children*. Mosby, St Louis, MO.

Prosser, S., Worster, B., MacGregor, J. *et al.* (2000) *Applied Pharmacology*. Mosby, London.

Sacks, O. (1995) *An Anthropologist on Mars*. Picador, London.

Websites

Acute confusional state: http://www.medical approaches.com
Epilepsy (self help): http://www.epilepsynse.org.uk

SELF-TEST QUESTIONS

Identify which of the following options are likely to apply. Some, all or none of the possible answers may be correct.

1. When a client who was previously lucid suddenly develops changes in their thought or behaviour patterns, the health professional should consider:
    a. instituting a programme of reality orientation
    b. whether a prescription for neuroleptic medication is needed
    c. whether a recent change in some aspect of the client's life has occurred
    d. getting a comprehensive assessment made of the client's physical health

2. A client has an assessment of her mental state and is found to score particularly badly in arithmetic calculation. This may be because:
    a. the client has never been good at numerical calculation
    b. medication has impaired her calculating ability
    c. the client was not given the reading glasses she usually uses
    d. an acute confusional state has impaired her ability to calculate

3. In acute confusional state a client's mental functioning may have changed because:
    a. he is suffering from age-related neuronal degeneration
    b. alterations in the composition of the extracellular fluid have impaired neuronal functioning
    c. there is a lack of available glucose for cerebral nutrition
    d. the thyroid gland is underactive

4. Which of the following neurotransmitters make neurones less excitable?
   a. acetylcholine
   b. serotonin
   c. dopamine
   d. gamma-aminobutyric acid
5. What is meant by the term 'seizure threshold'?
   a. the presence of raised pressure within the central nervous system
   b. the readiness of neurones to generate action potentials
   c. the ease with which positive ions can enter through the nerve cell membrane
   d. whether or not the client loses consciousness during a seizure
6. Which is the usual sequence of events in a tonic–clonic seizure?
   a. automatism; absence attack; loss of consciousness; confusion
   b. aura; absence attack; muscle pain; fatigue
   c. aura; localised limb jerking; confusion; drowsiness
   d. limb jerking during sleep
7. A client who has been recently diagnosed as having epilepsy is taking carbamazepine. He should be made aware that:
   a. he will need to have blood tests at intervals to assess the plasma levels of the drug
   b. it will be all right to continue taking his tricyclic antidepressants
   c. he should report any rashes and sore throats
   d. he can continue to take alcohol, as it will not interact with the drug
8. When a client has a tonic–clonic convulsion, her carers should:
   a. ensure that the airway remains clear in the tonic stage
   b. position the client on her side during the clonic stage
   c. allow privacy and rest during the postictal stage
   d. position the client on her side during the aura
9. Mental stress can cause physical illness because:
   a. the levels of neurotransmitters in the hypothalamus are depleted
   b. increased levels of corticosteroids diminish the activity of the immune system
   c. overactivity of the sympathetic nervous system may cause respiratory depression
   d. chronic elevation of the blood pressure may occur
10. A client is subject to hyperventilation attacks. He should be told that:
   a. the condition is harmless and self-limiting
   b. the tingling in his mouth can be controlled by breathing into a paper bag
   c. light-headedness is due to fatigue from the respiratory effort
   d. the chest pain he complains of is most probably due to indigestion

Answers

Chapter 1

Self-test questions
1. Options b. and c. are correct
2. All the statements are correct
3. Options a., c. and d. are correct
4. Option b. is correct
5. Options b. and d. are correct
6. Options a., c. and d. are correct
7. All the statements are correct
8. Options a., b., c. and d. are correct
9. Option b. is correct
10. Option d. is correct

Chapter 2

Case study 2.1 – Jess
1. Jess's doctor might have prescribed her a short dose of benzodiazepines to obtain rapid control of her symptoms, but there is a risk that the sudden relief of distressing symptoms could make her dependent on these agents, which is why a short prescription only would have been ordered. She has been prescribed a partial serotonin agonist, gepirone, which will slowly rebalance the levels of serotonin receptors at the synapses and gently bring the neural overstimulation under control.
2. The partial serotonin agonists interact less dramatically with alcohol than stronger sedative anxiolytics such as the benzodiazepines. However, Jess would be well advised to read the information leaflet that accompanies her tablets.

Case study 2.2 – Fergal
1. Fergal may have been given specific serotonin reuptake inhibitors (SSRIs), which can help sufferers from social phobia. They help to release inhibitions and reduce the fear of rejection that seems to be spoiling Fergal's life.
2. He might have been referred for an opinion as to whether he would benefit from cognitive behavioural therapy.

Case study 2.3 – Maggie
1. Maybe, maybe not. News reports about outbreaks of meningitis in schoolchildren might have played some part in it.

2. Biochemically, the condition is thought to be caused by an imbalance of the serotonin mechanisms, possibly also dopamine mechanisms. Maggie may receive a range of medications aimed at increasing the effectiveness of serotonin, including SSRIs, buspirone to slow consumption of serotonin at the synapses or serotonin partial agonists to increase the effectiveness of serotonin at the postsynaptic receptor. Medication is usually only part of the story. Maggie is likely to be offered some form of psychological treatment to expose her to her underlying fears and help her to acquire ways of coping with them. Modelling, in which someone she respects demonstrates to her appropriate cleaning strategies, may be used so that she relearns appropriate behaviours in relation to keeping the house clean.

3. Maggie should understand that the response to the medication is likely to be slow, about 8–12 weeks and is unlikely to be dramatic, so it would be useful to engage in the psychological therapy. If the SSRIs do not work, there are other drugs that can be added to her treatment regimen to augment the therapeutic effects.

Self-test questions

1. Options b. and d. are correct
2. Option c. is correct
3. All the statements are correct
4. Options b. and c. are correct
5. Options c. and d. are correct
6. All the statements are correct
7. Options a., c. and d. are correct
8. Options b. and c. are correct
9. Options b., c. and d. are correct. Ideally psychological therapy should accompany any pharmacological treatment. The use of bromocriptine would exacerbate the effects of OCD
10. Options a. and c. are correct

CHAPTER 3

Case study 3.1 – Thomas

1. The use of some recreational drugs can produce depression once the transient mood elevation has disappeared.
2. Fluoxetine has the side-effect of loss of libido. When he was depressed this would not have seemed to matter, as his sex drive was diminished anyway, but once another relationship developed it would have been problematic.
3. A dual reuptake inhibitor such as bupropion might have been helpful, as sexual function is relatively unaffected by this drug.

Case study 3.2 – Maxine

1. Tricyclics take a period of around 10 days to build up a therapeutic

concentration in the central nervous system and only then will the improvement in Maxine's mood become noticeable.

2. Maxine's depression is associated with anxiety, so SSRIs would tend to enhance these feelings. She might benefit from one of the newer dual reuptake inhibitors.

3. She may have blurring of vision, which can impede sustained reading of small print. This is one of the antimuscarinic effects of tricyclic antidepressants. The weight gain is likely to result from histamine receptor blockade, which interferes with weight control.

Case study 3.3 – Jason

1. At present Jason has no insight into his situation, and feels good, so is unlikely to find any lowering of his mood acceptable. He is unlikely to concentrate for long enough to accept an explanation but treatment may need to be instituted for his own good before he gets into serious problems through his excessive behaviour.

2. His bipolar disease could have been precipitated by neurostimulatory drugs, which some people use to enhance their mood and performance. Jason's current view of himself as a rock star may well stem from aspirations that would have been boosted by such substances.

3. Compounds such as carbamazepine, clozapine or sodium valproate may be used to reduce the level of activity of nerve cells and thus regulate his mood. The best established agent is lithium, although it is potentially toxic. Each of these agents has inherent hazards related to use, and potential drug interactions. There may be additional problems if Jason does indeed use recreational drugs.

Self-test questions

1. Options b. and d. are correct. Delusions and hallucinations do not form part of major depression
2. None of the options is correct
3. Options a., b. and c. are correct. Dysthymia is thought to be commoner in women than men
4. None of the options is correct
5. All the statements may be true
6. Options a., b. and c. are correct
7. Options c. and d. are correct
8. All the options are correct
9. All the statements are correct
10. All the statements are correct

CHAPTER 4

Case study 4.1 – Janice

1. 'Coming home' triggers binge eating in some people. Although we don't know this, Janice may have anxiety-related problems or

lowered self-esteem. Family factors may have contributed to her condition, or she might recently have left home and be missing a particular person. Although, again, we don't know this, she may also have pre-existing depression.

2. At the excessive doses she is taking, Janice is likely to put herself at risk of fluid and electrolyte imbalance, as well as causing herself physical discomfort. Purging or inducing vomiting are thought to be indicators of more severe types of bulimia nervosa.

3. As Janice binged over a period of some hours and a significant amount of her meal comprised 4 litres of ice cream, presumably eaten slowly with a small spoon, her gastric stretch receptors might not have sent signals of satiety to her brain. Within the brain itself, there may be a disorder of the serotonin and noradrenaline (norepinephrine) neurotransmitters that normally moderate eating.

4. Yes, but the problem is getting her to recognise this and seek it. The secrecy and organisation of the binge suggests that she might have been doing this for some time.

Case study 4.2 – Jacquetta

1. Young female gymnasts may lose their extreme lightness and flexibility as they approach puberty. Trying to excel in gymnastics may have led Jacquetta to control her weight to try to maintain her place in the gym squad. Her father may have fuelled her anxieties about weight gain in his keenness to see her succeed. Jacquetta seems to control her weight by obsessive diet and exercising, rather than by vomiting and purging: this is thought in some circles to be associated with a better prognosis in anorexia nervosa. The fashion for thinness and for clothes that rely on a slender frame for best effect increase the interest of Jacquetta, and possibly her friends, in weight control.

2. We must bear in mind that she knows what Jacquetta looks like and we don't. If Jacquetta is underweight, the history of intensive exercise and obsessive weight control, plus her past as a gymnast who didn't quite make the grade, are suggestive of anorexia nervosa. We would need to know her height and weight: if her body mass index is below 16 her nutritional state would give cause for concern.

3. Possibly, the college medical centre could become involved if Jacquetta's tutors were concerned about her overall health. If Jacquetta was significantly underweight such that she was nearing a state of starvation, she would need specialist referral. The first imperative would be to assess the nutritional risk and then if possible to create a trusting relationship so as to help Jacquetta review her regime of low-energy foods and high-energy workouts. It would be useful to know if she is menstruating normally. Such questions could be interpreted by Jacquetta as being intrusive into her personal privacy and would need to be approached with care. Without effective psychological care and support, Jacquetta could

decline to co-operate and sustained starvation might put her life at risk.

Self-test questions

1. Option b. is correct. Insulin is only secreted when there is enough glucose in the blood to allow it to be used by cells other than those in the brain. The homeostatic control of metabolism means that a missed meal, even at the end of the fasting stage of metabolism, will not produce measurable weight loss. Adrenaline (epinephrine) is a hormone that sustains the short-term physical response to challenge.
2. Options a., c. and d. are correct
3. Options a., b. and d. are correct. If the metabolic rate rises, energy usage may outstrip energy intake and result in weight loss
4. Option d. is correct. Bulimic people may throw away food without bingeing on it. Food used for binges tends to consist of a range of 'convenience' products.
5. All the statements are correct
6. All the statements are correct
7. Options a. and d. are correct
8. Options a. and d. are correct
9. All the statements are correct
10. Options a., b. and d. are correct. Although hypnotic preparations induce sleep, the stages of the sleep cycle are abnormal.

CHAPTER 5

Self-test questions

1. a
2. a
3. b
4. c
5. a
6. d
7. d
8. c
9. b
10. b
11. d
12. d
13. d

CHAPTER 6

Case study 6.1 – Mary

Mary is obviously experiencing memory impairment, or amnesia, as evidenced by her forgetfulness about locking the door. It is likely that

Mary is struggling more generally with her short-term memory deficit. It is common for people to cope with some short-term memory loss in the early stages of dementia. Many find ways to compensate and rely heavily on those around them. Mary's problems have become more apparent since the death of her husband. With increasing memory loss there is a tendency for individuals to confabulate or fill in gaps in their memory with plausible experiences.

Activities of daily living become difficult to manage with the advent of apraxias. Mary was previously very house-proud but as her dementia has progressed she has found it increasingly difficult to perform tasks she could once master. This is having a profound effect on her ability to care for herself. It is unlikely that she is feeding herself properly and she has become a danger to herself in the kitchen and around the home. She has on several occasions set fire to pans as a direct result of her increasing cognitive deficit. Mary is also neglecting her personal hygiene and as a result is increasingly at risk of developing infections. Urine tract infections are likely to further exacerbate her mental confusion and increase the risks to her health and safety.

The intervention of Mary's daughter has not been without problems. Mary's inability to understand her daughter's requests, known as receptive aphasia, and an apparent inability to recognise her daughter for who she is, known as visual agnosia, have made it very difficult for her daughter to gain access to the house and offer support. Mary has also developed psychiatric symptoms such as a delusional belief that her daughter is out to steal her money.

Given the nature of Mary's deterioration and lack of accessibility to her home, it is likely that Mary will need to go into hospital for assessment of her mental state. Based on this, plans for her future care can be formulated.

Self-test questions

1. a
2. c
3. b
4. T
5. d
6. b
7. T
8. c
9. F
10. b
11. b
12. a

CHAPTER 7

Case study 7.1 – Fred

1. Initially Fred became **intoxicated** very quickly by alcohol acting as a depressant of neuronal functioning. He enjoyed the effects he was experiencing, which acted to reinforce his use of alcohol. However, repeated use of alcohol led to the development of **tolerance**, so that he needed more of the drug to achieve the desired effect. Adaptation of receptors at the GABA receptor complex produced a state of physiological **dependence** on alcohol, whereby Fred could not stop drinking without experiencing the effects of **withdrawal**. Attempts to stop drinking suddenly and without support inevitably failed as a result of the withdrawal he experienced.

2. Despite a desire to stop drinking, prompted by a series of injuries and relationship problems, Fred could not achieve his goal without support. The support came by way of an alcohol service that provided a safe means by which he could detoxify from the alcohol. Chlordiazepoxide, a benzodiazepine, was used as a substitute for alcohol, since it binds with receptors at the same GABA receptor complex where alcohol has its effects. A reducing regime allowed Fred to detoxify from the alcohol in a controlled manner and without the withdrawal effects he had experienced previously.

3. While Fred successfully underwent a detoxification from alcohol, and remained abstinent for a short time, he quickly returned to drinking large amounts of alcohol. This is common among this group and gives credence to the belief that tolerance and dependence are not the core of addiction. Detoxification in isolation rarely, if ever, forms a treatment plan for addiction. People who become dependent on alcohol need much greater levels of support if they are to achieve their goal of abstinence. Many forms of support are available, such as the 12-step process advocated by Alcoholics Anonymous. Additional support, when appropriate, can also be offered pharmacologically. This generally takes the form of medications that act as deterrents to drinking alcohol, such as disulfiram, and anti-craving medications such as naltrexone or acamprosate.

Self-test questions

1. b
2. b
3. c
4. c
5. d
6. T
7. a
8. b

9. b
10. d
11. a
12. d

CHAPTER 8

Case study 8.1 – Mr Patel

1. Dehydration, if sufficiently severe, will alter the osmolarity of tissue fluids, including those within the brain, even though the central nervous system is protected from sudden chemical shifts by the presence of the blood–brain barrier. This alters the movement of electrolytes across the cell membrane of the neurone and therefore influences the patterns of nerve transmission. If the neurone becomes hyperexcitable, then a confusional state may develop.

2. The confusional state developed over a short period of time. Investigation revealed that there was an organic disorder, which was then treated, and Mr Patel's cognitive function subsequently made a dramatic improvement, which is unlikely to have happened if he had had Alzheimer's disease.

3. The viral pneumonia would be likely to cause inflammation of the alveoli and small bronchioles, and thus would impair diffusion of oxygen into the blood, putting Mr Patel at risk of developing cerebral hypoxia. The brain is dependent on oxygen for cellular metabolism, if hypoxia occurs, then normal neural functioning is impaired and confusion may result.

Case study 8.2 – Peter

1. During the 'aura' (the illusory smell of frying bacon, perhaps), they might have noticed that Peter was behaving differently and might have helped him to put himself in a place of safety, away from the carpentry tools. During the tonic stage, they should have removed any hazardous objects in readiness for the clonic stage, when he might have knocked into heavy equipment, causing himself damage. In general, they should have tried to ensure that he was safe and avoided undue exposure during the attack. Following this, as the seizure settled, Peter would have been left to sleep in privacy and dignity. If he had been incontinent during the seizure, he might have appreciated help to change some of his clothing.

2. Obviously it is important that Peter enjoys as normal a life as possible. However, he must know that alcohol and anticonvulsant drugs often do not mix, so he might prefer to take alcohol-free drinks that are indistinguishable in appearance from the 'real thing'.

3. Peter may need his plasma drug levels to be checked: if these are moving out of the therapeutic range (above or below), then this may cause an increase in frequency of the seizures. It would be

important to check that he is not taking any other non-prescribed medication that might interact with his anticonvulsants, induce liver enzymes and cause untoward drug reactions.

Case study 8.3 – Joan

1. Joan needs to know that the hyperventilation is at the root of her spiralling symptoms. An attack is commonly triggered either by an emotional stimulus or sometimes by increased release of metabolic acids by the tissues. The dizziness and lightheadedness are probably the outcome of reduction of carbon dioxide levels in the blood, which causes the acid–base balance to be disturbed and the plasma to become alkalotic. This eventually alters the chemistry in the cranial cavity, causing the symptoms. It can often be demonstrated to clients that, if they rebreathe into a paper bag, thus increasing their carbon dioxide levels, their symptoms improve and the vicious circle is broken. The numbness around the mouth and the sensation in the chest are also due to the altered chemistry and will improve if the hyperventilation can be interrupted.

2. Chronic hyperventilation is thought to cause narrowing of blood vessels in the coronary and cerebral circulations. Systemic hypertension and myocardial ischaemia or infarction may subsequently result, although the way this should be conveyed to an already anxious patient requires careful thought.

3. A beta-adrenergic blocker such as propranolol may be helpful as it will suppress the sense of anxiety as well as reducing symptoms associated with activation of the sympathetic nervous system.

Case study 8.4 – Halma and Miss Spinks

1. Halma's symptoms are consistent with an overactive thyroid.

2. Thyroid hormones increase the metabolic rate. This produces an overall increase in energy needs, resulting in increased appetite and weight loss. Increased metabolism in the central nervous system results in heightened neuromuscular tone, hence the tremor; and increased mental activity, hence the hyperactivity and tendency to anxiety.

3. In summary: eventually the metabolic rate in the tissues increases to such an extent that the cardiovascular system fails to meet the metabolic needs of the tissues – so-called high-output cardiac failure, which may be lethal.

4. Miss Spinks's symptoms are consistent with underactivity of the thyroid gland.

5. The main risk associated with untreated underactivity of the thyroid gland is of hypothermia due to the reduced heat production resulting from a lower than normal metabolic rate. Miss Spinks would also be at risk of developing myxoedema, which, in summary, could proceed to myxoedemic coma and subsequently death.

6. Hypothyroidism produces a generalised slowing down of metabolic

processes. Thus, in essence, the person suffers a generalised slowing of all processes: speech, mental processes, general activity levels, eating and elimination are all retarded, which may present a similar picture to that of the patient with significant clinical depression, or certain types of dementia. In addition, untreated hypothyroidism can produce a psychotic condition known as 'myxoedema madness'.

Self-test questions

1. Options c. and d. are correct, as sudden changes in cognition and behaviour may be caused by an acute confusional state.
2. All the options are correct
3. Options b. and c. are correct. Age-related degeneration in itself is not a cause of acute confusional state, although the degenerative process may make the client more vulnerable to the development of acute confusional state. Thyroid underactivity may cause dementia sometimes, but not acute confusional state.
4. Options a. and d. are correct. Serotonin and dopamine are usually excitatory neurotransmitters
5. Options b. and c. are correct
6. None of the options are correct
7. Options a. and c. are correct. Carbamazepine and tricyclic antidepressants or alcohol can interact, producing an adverse reaction.
8. Option c. is correct. Rigidity of the jaw muscle makes it unwise to try to open the mouth to ensure that the airway is clear; during the clonic stage, violent limb movements make it impossible to position or maintain the person in the recovery position. During the aura, the patient is conscious but may put him- or herself in a place of safety in anticipation of the impending convulsion.
9. Options b. and d. are correct. Overactivity of the sympathetic nervous system would cause increased respiratory effort to be made.
10. Option b. is correct. Rebreathing the expired air will cause a gradual increase of carbon dioxide levels in the blood and will return the blood acidity levels to healthy values. Untreated chronic hyperventilation may cause harmful changes to vasculature in the brain and coronary circulation and may result in the development of coronary artery insufficiency or hypertension. Light-headedness does occur but the cause is altered chemistry of the tissue fluid in the brain, not respiratory fatigue. Chest pain may be due to indigestion but it also may be caused by angina pectoris: pain due to insufficient circulation to the heart muscle.

INDEX